Sex, Gay Men and AIDS

Peter M. Davies, Ford C.I. Hickson,
Peter Weatherburn and Andrew J. Hunt

with

Paul J. Broderick, Tony P.M. Coxon,
Tom J. McManus and Michael J. Stephens

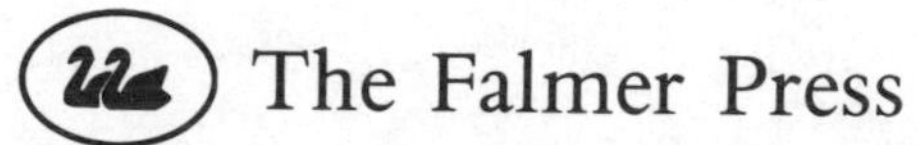

The Falmer Press
(A member of the Taylor & Francis Group)
London · New York · Philadelphia

UK The Falmer Press, 4 John St, London WC1N 2ET
USA The Falmer Press, Taylor & Francis Inc., 1900 Frost Road, Suite 101, Bristol, PA 19007

First published 1993

A catalogue record for this book is available from the British Library

ISBN 0 75070 095 5
ISBN 0 75070 096 3 pbk

Typeset in 9.5/11 Bembo
by Graphicraft Typesetters Ltd, Hong Kong

Printed in Great Britain by Burgess Science Press, Basingstoke on paper which has a specified pH value on final paper manufacture of not less than 7.5 and is therefore 'acid free'.

This volume is dedicated
to the memory of
ANDREW HUNT
Senior Researcher on Project SIGMA
Who died on Christmas Day, 1992

Contents

Series Editor's Preface

Since the earliest days of the epidemic it has been claimed that an understanding of sexual behaviour is essential to the development of effective approaches to HIV prevention. Nowhere is this more true than in relation to sex between men, given that in many developed countries gay and bisexual men continue to be at greatest risk of infection. But an adequate appreciation of the nature of male homosexual practice and desire must move beyond a number of unhelpful and divisive 'theories' about the origins and nature of that which is to be explained — most particularly those which would have us understand sex between men as something unusual or unnatural: a gross moral turpitude or a sickness to be cured. For such narratives too frequently misread the phenomenon to be explained; constructing gay men, or 'homosexuals' as they are more usually called, artificially, monolithically and in subordinate relation to dominant heterosexual norms.

Drawing on data from Project SIGMA, the first British in-depth study of sex, gay men and HIV/AIDS, this book offers a cogent critique of unhelpful stereotypes and outdated theories and assumptions such as these. It provides new insight into the nature of sexual activity between men, transcending the individualism and negativism implicit in earlier accounts. Certain to become a standard source of reference in years to come, and crucial reading for policy-makers, health educators and activists alike, *Sex, Gay Men and AIDS* offers a more thoroughgoing analysis of the epidemic and its effects than has hitherto been possible.

Peter Aggleton

Preface

That this is a joint production can easily be seen from the list of authors, yet many more people have contributed to this volume than are named there. To these, we owe a debt of gratitude which we here acknowledge. First, we would like to thank our respondents who have given liberally of their time and hospitality and of the intimate and intricate details of their most private lives. This is, in a very real sense, their book. We would also like to thank all those who over the last five years have worked for or with Project SIGMA. We would like especially to thank Clive Rees, Mike Millington, Gerard Phillips, Adrian Coyle, Rory Murray and Paul Simpson, who, as part of the original research team, all worked hard to put together the original cohort. We also thank Malcolm Macourt, who ran the Newcastle office, and Sheena Sutherland, without whose hard work the seroprevalence study would not have been possible.

We have a debt of gratitude to those at South Bank Polytechnic (now University) who supported our efforts in an institution whose attitude to our research was, at best, equivocal. Those included Miriam David and other members of the now defunct Department of Social Sciences, Ian Sillett and Gerard Chick of the Industrial Liaison Unit and Lil Brown of the Finance Department. Similar thanks are due to some members of the Sociology Department, University College Cardiff (later University of Wales, College of Cardiff), especially Sara Delamount and Paul Atkinson, and Jenny Morgan of the Occupational Health Unit.

We record our indebtedness to the funding authorities, the Medical Research Council and the Department of Health (formerly the Department of Health and Social Security). We particularly thank Anne Kauder and Liza Catan of the AIDS Unit at the Department of Health for help and guidance beyond the call of duty.

In addition to those already mentioned, and the current team members, all the following have contributed to this book by working with or for SIGMA at some point in the last six years or so: Phillip Attwood, Scott Beveridge, Theo Blackmore, Terry Blair, David Blenkinsop, Anthony Brand, Alan Burnside, Paul Calander, George Christofinis, Huw Coxon, David Cumberland, Chris Davies, Scott Dawson, Nigel Foote, John Gay, Michael Gray, Pat Holland, Adrian Jacobs, Angela Jones, Barry Jones, Simon Jones, Vijay Kumari, David Langley, Philip Looker, Deborah Lowry, Kathy Marshall, Helen Moore, Patrick Price, David Pye, Alan Quirk, Sue Radford, Omar Rey, Dominic Riley, Siân Roberts, Lynda

Ryder, Tony Shannon, Margaret Simpson, Martin Simpson, Keri Summers, Glenn Townsend, Nikki Tragen, Patricia Wallace, Steven Walton and Gary Wych.

This preface already begins to resemble the egregious fulsomeness of the award recipient; to avoid any further deterioration in that direction, we would like not to thank our partners, parents, friends and pets. Suffice it to say that if any thanks was due, it has been given already.

Despite the contributions of all those above and those whom faulty memory or other reasons have omitted, the ideas and interpretations contained in this book are those of the authors.

Peter M. Davies, Ford C.I. Hickson, Peter Weatherburn and Andrew J. Hunt

1 Introduction and Overview

In 1948 Alfred Kinsey and his colleagues published a volume, expansively titled *Sexual Behaviour in the Human Male*. The overarching universality of the title belied the narrow range of men whose accounts formed the basis of the volume and occasioned some comment at the time. Similarly, the title of this book owes more to its fortunate congruence with the project's title than to any claim to be a universally valid, exactly definitive, account of sex, gay men and HIV. Nevertheless, since 1987, 1083 men have taken part in this study, entitled Socio-sexual Investigation of Gay Men and AIDS (hereafter SIGMA). All have been interviewed at least once, some up to four times, making a total of 2520 interviews, taking approximately 5500 hours. This makes Project SIGMA one of the largest and most detailed studies of male homosexual behaviour ever undertaken.

In this volume we have sought to provide a description of sexual mores among gay and bisexual men in England and Wales in the period 1987 to 1991, a time which has to be recognised as the time of AIDS. In this our focus has been rather broader than the narrow concerns of much current AIDS literature. We firmly believe that an account of safer sexual behaviour in the age of HIV and AIDS needs to be grounded in a theory of sexual behaviour in general: a point which much AIDS literature ignores. In doing so, we find ourselves drawn closer to the (fragile) tradition of British empirical research into male homosexuality, particularly the humane and comprehensive work of Michael Schofield, our most recent predecessor (see Chapter 2), than to many of our colleagues who specialise in HIV prevention. As a consequence, we have found ourselves concentrating more closely on providing what we regard as a compelling account of sexual behaviour which incorporates safer sex, than engaging directly with many of the current debates in the AIDS literature. We have published our critical contributions to these debates in the journals devoted to such matters.

Conversely, we believe that this book does directly address many of the problems of safer sex that are side-stepped or ignored by the traditional approaches. Moreover, we seek to do this by locating concerns about HIV in a wider context, as do the men we have talked to at some length. It is easy for AIDS professionals such as ourselves to see in safer sex the single most important issue in the gay community, the country or the world according to scope and preference. For us and them, it is a pervasive and ever present concern. Yet for many gay men, most of the time, it is not an important concern. However, it is also undeniable that

AIDS has affected *all* gay and bisexual men in Britain to some extent. This book seeks to capture the dimensions of response to that acquaintance.

How to Cheat When Reading This Book

The next three chapters (2, 3 and 4) provide the background to our work. Chapter 2 begins by charting the history of research into homosexuality in this country from the turn of the century. We seek to isolate some of the themes, debates and discourses that inform our personal and societal responses to AIDS. Chapter 3 gives a brief chronological account of the impact of HIV on gay and bisexual men in Britain in the 1980s, while Chapter 4 introduces some of the metaphorical constructions that have informed responses to this impact.

The following three chapters (5, 6 and 7) describe the specific context of and background to our research. The general reader may omit most of this section on first reading and treat it as a reference resource. Readers so minded, should, however, read Chapter 5 and the first two sections of Chapter 6 in order to understand our perspective. Chapter 6 describes and justifies the methods used by the project in obtaining and interpreting data. It seeks also to be honest about the shortcomings of the data. Chapter 7 provides a detailed breakdown of the characteristics of the respondents in the four waves of the study.

The next four chapters (8, 9, 10 and 11) form the substantive heart of the book and concentrate directly on sexual behaviour and organisation in the light of HIV. A brief account of the issues surrounding HIV antibody testing, as described by our respondents, and the data on seroprevalence that the project obtained are given in Chapter 8. Chapter 9 charts some of the individual parameters on sexual behaviour with men and women: incidence and frequencies of sexual techniques, numbers of sexual partners and other matters. Chapter 10 discusses at length the varied understandings that gay and bisexual men have of anal intercourse, the single sexual act most implicated in the transmission of HIV between men. Chapter 11 seeks to show how these understandings are used, together with existing patterns of sexual partnership, to create a strategic approach to safer sex.

The short final chapter sketches some broad conclusions and implications of the research.

The Use of Language

We construct, constrain and control our experience through and within language. Talking about the world confers and conveys our mastery of it. Towards the end of the nineteenth century a new vocabulary was created to talk about deviant sexualities. This was a vocabulary and a discourse designed to limit discussion of these heady matters to the educated few: the medical and judicial elites, or, at least, those who had facility in Latin. While the practice of writing on matters sexual in foreign or dead languages has thankfully disappeared, there remains a fastidiousness about robust vocabulary which threatens to restrict discussion to the educated. As we note in Chapter 6, we were at pains when interviewing the men involved in this study to use the vocabulary they chose and felt most comfortable using. Almost all choose to speak of their sexual experiences using 'street' terms, the earthy but robust vernacular. We feel that to speak of these experiences, to relay their ideas using a 'high' language, would be to betray and distance ourselves from the real world in which they, and we, live. We have chosen therefore to use, where appropriate, street terms.

2 Historical Background

> This is the first point to grasp about the history of this people. [The country] is impossible. [It] exists only because the [people] invented it. [They] exist only because they invented themselves. They had no choice. (G.A. Williams)

Despite its specific concern with male homosexual behaviour under the impact of AIDS, this volume stands in a fragile and fragmented British tradition of research into male homosexuality which reaches back almost exactly a century. In that time the meanings attached to male homosexual behaviour have changed dramatically more than once. To speak, as we do today, of homosexual individuals would have been quite incomprehensible little more than a century ago. The notion that individuals might be arrayed along a spectrum of hetero-homosexual experience was outrageous when it was put forward in the 1940s. The revolutionary proclamation of gay pride in the 1970s was breathtaking in its audacity. These contributions, together with many others, form a matrix within which this current volume was formed and without which it could not have existed. Equally, it is important to situate the responses of gay and bisexual men to AIDS in the 1980s in a very specific historical moment. It is impossible to appreciate the range and complexity of gay men's responses without some understanding of the community which produced and nurtured them. It is equally impossible to understand the political preoccupations of the gay community with regard to testing, treatment and access to health care without an appreciation of the historical relationship between the communities and the medical profession.

In this first two chapters of this book we seek to provide an outline of the historical and social context within which our work is situated. It would be unfeasible to provide in such a short space an exhaustive history, so we confine ourselves to a modest aim. In this first chapter we concentrate on the role of empirical research in defining the gay experience in the twentieth century and we aim, furthermore, to do so from a narrow British perspective, commenting on events elsewhere only when they are indispensable. In the second chapter we outline the history of AIDS in Great Britain from our (partial) perspective.

'Sexual Inversion'

In 1897 Havelock Ellis published the first volume of his *Studies in the Psychology of Sex*, a volume entitled *Sexual Inversion*, dealing with what we would now term homosexuality.[1] Broadly, Ellis was concerned with the humane project which in the late nineteenth century began to describe the homosexual individual, that is a person with a specific sexual attraction towards persons of the same gender. Since this notion has in the intervening century become so taken for granted, it is sometimes difficult to discard the idea and reconstruct the climate in which the suggestion was so revolutionary. According to recent scholarship, dating from McIntosh (1968) and Foucault (1979), the dominant idea before the latter half of the nineteenth century was that all individuals were capable of and tempted to homosexual acts in the same way that all are capable of and tempted to theft. Engaging in either was, then, evidence of wickedness.

By contrast, writers in the late nineteenth century began to describe a small group of defective individuals who were, for some reason, homosexual by nature. This revolutionary formulation forms part of the positivist challenge of the late nineteenth century, which sought the causes of anti-social behaviour in the genetic, somatic or psychological makeup of the individual. Ideas about the specific causes of homosexuality varied. There were those like Freud who regarded it as the outcome of a defective upbringing. Others, amongst whom Ellis is numbered, were more drawn to a genetic explanation.

Havelock Ellis was one of the last Victorians, a man of solitary temperament and immense industry, whose task it became to describe the vagaries of human sexual diversity. In this undertaking he shared the great Victorian impulse to collect, label and classify: the impulse that has bequeathed us the museums of South Kensington and works such as *The Golden Bough*. In his treatment of the subject Ellis distinguishes between homosexuality which is an empirical feature of sexual behaviour (this or that sexual encounter is homosexual or not depending on the gender of those involved) and what he terms sexual inversion, which he defines as: 'Sexual inversion, as here understood means sexual instinct turned by inborn constitutional abnormality towards persons of the same sex' (quoted in Grosskurth, 1980: 185). The distinction between an invert, someone who is 'born that way', and a 'pervert', someone who is capable of 'normal' response but who chooses homosexual activity, is basic to Ellis' argument. In the last analysis he disapproves of the latter but is prepared to condone the former.

Like his influential German contemporary, Richard von Krafft-Ebing, whose major work, *Psychopathia Sexualis*, was first published in English in 1892, Ellis uses case histories as evidence in this project. They differ in that Krafft-Ebing was concerned to establish the aetiology of sexual dysfunction as a step towards cure, and regarded most sexual 'abnormalities' as evidence of moral degeneracy (mostly caused by masturbation), while Ellis' concerns ran in rather different channels.

The evidence for this 'inborn constitutional abnormality' is, it must be said, weak in Ellis' account. His evidence is the strength of the sexual drive, the tendency for inversion to run in families and its early appearance (around the age of 9) (Rowbotham and Weeks, 1977: 158). Nevertheless, having established to his satisfaction the congenital nature of inversion, Ellis moves to impugn contemporary condemnations of homosexuality by pointing to other periods of European history and other contemporary cultures where such condemnations do not occur. As Weeks (Rowbotham and Weeks, 1977: 156) has pointed out: 'The two principles he employed were a form of cultural relativism as applied to moral attitudes and biological determinism as applied to essential sexual characteristics.' This approach allows him to assert that, (i) since inversion is inborn, deeply rooted in the psyche and amenable to change only with great difficulty and (ii) since other cultures have allowed homosexual expression without catastrophe, then (iii) it follows that inverted individuals deserve sympathy rather than condemnation. Ellis is, of course, open to convincing challenge on each and every part of this formulation and few today would make these arguments precisely in these terms, yet his influence is important for two main reasons. First, and very specifically, the broad thrust of the argument underpins the liberal view which guided the Wolfenden Committee and led, eventually, to the Sexual Offences Act of 1967, which to this day governs male homosexual behaviour in the UK. Second, while few of Ellis' ideas have had the longevity or wide ranging impact of another of his contemporaries, Freud, whose works he introduced to this country, he remains an influential British figure in the creation of the homosexual individual as a focus of medical, scientific and public attention. This is a complex process which has a number of consequential, though sometimes paradoxical features.

First, it allows and encourages the pathologising of the homosexual individual and the attendant search for the cause(s) of homosexuality and the associated cure (see Bullough, 1974). The move from homosexual acts to the homosexual individual has been characterised as moving 'from sin to sickness'. The homosexual individual becomes an object of scientific curiosity, and the list of 'cures' that have been inflicted on individuals in the pursuit of humanity and in the name of science is long and inglorious (see Weinberg, 1973).

Second, by naming a type of person, it shifts the ground of the moral debate. As long as homosexual acts were equally seductive to all individuals and chosen only by some, then those who were weak enough to succumb were guilty of a moral, more or less rational choice, for which society exacted condign punishment. To the extent, by contrast, that the individual is congenitally predisposed towards homosexual desire and acts, then to that extent the choice becomes one for which sympathy and treatment rather than opprobrium and punishment become appropriate.

Third, and in many ways paradoxically, the move from acts to identity allows the possibility of individual pride and community solidarity. It is no accident that at the same time as the homosexual individual was being created as an object of scientific discourse, a lawyer from Hanover, Karl Heinrich Ulrichs (Kennedy, 1988), was creating what is, arguably, the first modern homosexual liberation movement. Using arguments which rely on the new understanding of the homosexual individual, Ulrichs aimed to establish the naturalness of homosexual desire and the consequent right to what we would now term human rights. Other writers, notably the 'bard of Brooklyn', the American poet, Walt Whitman, sought, in the glorious camaraderie and ignoble slaughter of the American Civil War a language of homoerotic desire which broke from the constraints of moralistic censure. Others such as John Addington Symonds (1983) sought to claim classical precedent in the works of Plato for their conception of homosexual love as a refined, spiritual, transcendental experience. It is this tradition to which Oscar

Wilde had recourse when, at his trial in 1895, he was asked to describe 'the love that dare not speak its name'. He said:

> The 'Love that dare not speak its name' in this country is such a great affection of an elder for a younger man as there was between David and Jonathon, such as Plato made the very basis of his philosophy and such as you find in the sonnets of Michaelangelo and Shakespeare. It is that deep, spiritual affection that is pure as it is perfect. It dictates and pervades great works of art like those of Shakespeare and Michaelangelo, and those two letters of mine, such as they are. . . . It is beautiful, it is fine, it is the noblest form of affection. There is nothing unnatural about it. It is intellectual and it repeatedly exists between an elder and a younger man, where the elder has intellect and the younger has all the joy, hope and glamour of life before him. That it should be so, the world does not understand. The world mocks at it and sometimes puts one in the pillory for it. (quoted in Ellman, 1987: 435)

Dimensions of Homosexual Experience

In 1938 an obscure professor of biology at Indiana University, Alfred C. Kinsey, was asked, for reasons which remain obscure, according to his biographer (Pomeroy, 1972: 52), to coordinate a course on 'marriage', which was to involve contributions from a range of disciplines. The course was one of a number on the subject that were being set up in the more progressive universities in America and in Britain and typically included information on the biology of reproduction and, in a few cases, information on birth control. Kinsey's interest in human sexual behaviour developed as a result of this course and led to the publication of his enormously influential volumes on the male (1948) and the female (1953).

Alfred Kinsey's classic work on male sexual practices is firmly within that tradition of social research that applies the methods and procedures of natural science to the social world. Indeed, it has been remarked that Kinsey's methodology in his work on the gall wasp (1942) did not differ significantly from that in his work on sexual behaviour. In his determined empiricism Kinsey reflected the outlook of contemporary American science but also shared the same naturalistic premises and devotion to collecting data as Ellis. By studying sexual behaviour as an empirical 'fact', Kinsey could only, strictly, establish what is the case. But he recognised, as did many of his contemporaries, that these empirical data would also profoundly influence moral debate, debate about what ought to be the case.

In the pursuit (or as some would have it, the vain hope) of objectivity, Kinsey concentrated exclusively on the (reported) incidence of orgasm in his sample (Kinsey *et al.*, 1948: 193) and largely ignored the thorny questions of identity, opportunity and social construction that surround and pervade the subject. In so doing, he provided a mass of data that has served as a baseline for a host of subsequent studies and interpretations and policy initiatives. Indeed, we commented in 1986:

> It is symptomatic of this dearth of information that those figures most often quoted for the incidence of homosexual behaviour (Kinsey *et al.*, 1948) are fifty years old, relate only to the white population of the United

> States and are known to embody major errors and biases (Cochran *et al.*, 1954). Nevertheless, a whole range of policy decisions, involving millions of pounds of future and present expenditure is based on the flimsiest of evidence and the most cursory acquaintance with homosexual men and their lifestyles. (Davies, 1986: 1)

Specifically with regard to homosexual behaviour, the study has proved seminal for two main contributions. First, it revealed that the incidence of homosexual behaviour was much greater than had hitherto been supposed. Counting only homosexual relations to the point of orgasm, he writes:

> [t]he data in the present study indicate that at least 37% of the male population has some homosexual experience between the beginning of adolescence and old age. This is more than one male in three of the persons that one may meet as he passes along the street. Among the males who remain unmarried to the age of 35, almost exactly 50% have homosexual experience. . . . These figures are, of course, considerably higher than any which have previously been estimated; but . . . they must be understatements, if they are anything other than fact. (pp. 623–5)

Second, he suggested that men could be arranged along a continuum of sexual response, moving from those who are completely heterosexual in their behaviour, to whom he gave a 'score' of 0, through varying degrees of mixed heterosexual-homosexual response to those who are completely homosexual, to whom he gave a 'score' of 6. It is not clear whether a seven-point scale is preferable to one with any other number of grades in dividing up this continuum, and indeed Kinsey specifically refers to gradations within each of the categories (p. 647), but the labelling has entered into the realm of common knowledge (a popular T-shirt slogan of several years ago read 'Kinsey 6'). Kinsey wrote pungently:

> Males do not represent two discrete populations, heterosexual and homosexual. The world is not divided into sheep and goats. Not all things are black nor all things white. . . . Only the human mind invents categories and tries to force facts into separated pigeonholes. The living world is a continuum in each and every one of its aspects. The sooner we learn this concerning human sexual behaviour, the sooner we shall reach a sound understanding of the realities of sex. (p. 639)

It would be easy, and a little unfair, to criticise the 'sheep and goats' distinction between cognitive categories and facts in this formulation, but the important point that he made has yet to reach those who blithely suppose a hermetic gay community, separate from the heterosexual, within which HIV can be contained without undue concern (see Chapter 3).

It is worth reiterating Kinsey's summative generalisations (pp. 650–1) on the incidence of homosexual behaviour if only to be clear about exactly what the study did show. He records that in the white population as covered by his study:

> 37% of the total male population have at least some overt homosexual experience to the point of orgasm between adolescence and old age.

50% of the males who remain single until age 35 have had overt homosexual experience to the point of orgasm since the onset of adolescence.

63% of all males never have overt homosexual experience to the point of orgasm after the onset of adolescence.

13% of males (approximately) react erotically to other males without having overt homosexual contacts after the onset of adolescence.

30% of all males have at least incidental homosexual experience or reactions over at least a three-year period between the ages of 16 and 55.

25% of the male population have more than incidental homosexual experience or reactions for at least three years between the ages of 16 and 55.

18% of the males have at least as much of the homosexual as the heterosexual in their histories.

13% of the population have more of the homosexual than the heterosexual for at least three years between the ages of 16 and 55.

10% of the males are more or less exclusively homosexual for at least three years between the ages of 16 and 55.

8% of the males are exclusively homosexual for at least three years between 16 and 55.

4% of the white males are exclusively homosexual throughout their lives after the onset of adolescence.

It should be apparent from this range of data that the question, 'who is homosexual?', has no one, clear answer and that the population that is of interest in a study of the homosexual experience ranges (on these figures) from approximately 1.1 million men in the UK to approximately 12.5 million. It should also be pointed out to those gay activists who blithely assert that 10% of the population is (or, in some versions, could be if they tried) homosexual and that the figure was established by Kinsey, that this is not the case. Indeed, the figure of 10% has no sustainable claim to validity and should be quietly abandoned by those who seek to establish the case for equality on the basis of statistics.

In the same way that the establishment of the 'homosexual' as an object of scientific curiosity in the 1860s was paralleled by the formation of the first modern homosexual emancipation movement, so the publication of the Kinsey report coincided with the founding of the Mattachine Society in California, the direct precursor of the gay liberation movements of the late 1960s and 1970s. The name is said to derive from one of the medieval French *sociétés joyeux*, called the *Société Mattachine* (Katz, 1976, p. 620). These societies, according to the founder of Mattachine, Harry Hay, were, '. . . lifelong secret fraternities of unmarried townsmen who never performed in public unmasked, were dedicated to going into the countryside and conducting dances and rituals during the Feast of Fools, at the Vernal Equinox' (p. 621). Though by no means the first society of its type, its founding was symptomatic of a recrudescence of the sense of community and struggle, built, it has been suggested (Bérubé, 1983; d'Emilio, 1983), by the experiences of homosexual men and women in the forces during the 1939–45 war. Although homosexual acts remained illegal in the Allied armed forces, the male bonding that was a powerful feature of life in the forces created a situation where many could explore the homosocial and, clandestinely, the homosexual aspects of their lives. It has been suggested (Kaye Wellings, personal communication) that the 'high' figures for male homosexual contact recorded by Kinsey are due, at least in part, to the fact that the study took place in the war years.

The Liberal Consensus

Almost ten years after the publication of Kinsey, the Wolfenden Committee (Home Office/Scottish Home Department, 1957) stated, with its usual, exasperating even-handedness: 'Some of us have the definite impression . . . that there has been an increase in the amount of homosexual behaviour. Others of us prefer . . . not to commit ourselves to expressing even a general impression' (para. 44). As evidence of this increase (if, indeed, it had occurred), the committee cited the 'general loosening of former moral standards', 'the conditions of wartime and the prolonged separation of the sexes', which might have occasioned 'homosexual behaviour which in some cases has been carried over into peacetime' and 'emotional insecurity, community instability and weakening of the family' (para. 45). Nevertheless, they remark that Kinsey's estimates of the incidence of homosexuality, in the opinion of their medical witnesses, 'would be on the high side for Great Britain' (para. 38), and they cite favourably a Swedish survey (para. 39) suggesting an incidence of just 1% exclusively homosexual (compared with Kinsey's 4%).

The Wolfenden Committee's report was among the most important of a series of publications in the 1950s and 1960s which created the groundswell of middle-class opinion which eventually allowed the passing of the 1967 Sexual Offences Act. These works came either from 'concerned liberals' (e.g., Magee, 1966; Chesser, 1959; Westwood, 1952, 1960; Hauser, 1962) or from 'self-confessed' homosexuals (Plummer, 1963; Cory, 1953; Cory and Leroy, 1963).

The philosophical stance of these works was, in general, liberal; that is, the tone is one of tolerance rather than acceptance. This was predicated on two notions, which do not always sit as neatly together as we might wish. First, they accepted that certain individuals are fated to be homosexual by inclination. Most texts therefore feature a discussion of the aetiology of homosexuality, and while Ellis' ideas of genetic causation and the evidence from twin studies, for example, are cited, most writers veer towards belief in an acquired trait. For example, West (1955: 15) writes, 'Exclusive preference for the opposite sex is an acquired trait and involves the repression of a certain amount of homosexual feeling which is natural to the human being. . . . On the other hand, the completely homosexual man, one who is repelled rather than attracted by feminine charms, really suffers from an abnormal inhibition, the origin of which can often be traced to psychological causes early in life.' The key to the argument lies, however, in the propositions that, whatever the exact aetiology, the homosexual inclination was relatively fixed and the result of genetic inheritance or events in early childhood. From this premise, a tranche of arguments could be made for sympathetic treatment. Homosexuality was more an illness or a handicap than a crime and, as such, those afflicted (the terminology is indicative) were deserving more of sympathy than of condemnation. As an illness, of course, the possibility of cure was theoretically present; and though the current attempts were not very successful, writers were at pains to stress that they were not encouraging men to be or become homosexual. On the contrary,

> The fact that many young men grow out of homosexual habits as they get older casts doubt on the assumption that sexual orientation is always firmly fixed either in childhood or in youth. No doubt, some individuals are doomed from infancy . . . but others remain potentially capable of heterosexual development even in their twenties. The comparatively hopeless cases, for whom no known treatment holds out much hope of change, are older persons who have practised homosexuality for years and have never tried, or wanted to try, to function heterosexually. (West, 1955: 266)

On the other hand, the Freudian proposition that homosexual attraction is universal but that some individuals were more successful than others in repressing it and leading 'normal' lives, fitted well with Kinsey's astounding figures for the incidence of homosexual behaviour. Westwood comments: 'If the laws relating to homosexuality were rigidly enforced, over one in three of the total male population would have to be segregated from the rest' (Westwood, 1952: 164). And what fun that could be!

Since the number of men convicted of homosexual offences was far lower than this, it followed that many homosexuals lived more or less productive lives despite this handicap. Furthermore, a case could be made for regarding some of the great figures of Western culture as homosexual. The question arose of the role of the law in the control of homosexual behaviour. The emergent view was that the law was counter-productive and inappropriate. As Westwood noted: 'The laws were made and passed many years before the true nature of the homosexual impulse was understood. What we now know is a serious mental disease was considered to be a vice and a crime in those days' (Westwood, 1952: 164).

It is possible to regard the consensus that emerged in the liberal middle class — what came to be known as the 'chattering classes' — during the 1950s and 1960s was a reversion to a pre-positivist view of homosexuality. In both cases homosexual behaviour is a potential for all individuals. In the earlier version the choice was a moral one, whereas in the more modern view genetic inheritance or deficient upbringing predisposed some more than others. The Wolfenden Committee put their collective finger accurately on the essential similarity of these two views, despite their apparent difference: 'There is no *prima facie* grounds for supposing that because a particular person's sexual propensity happens to lie in the direction of persons of his or her own sex it is any less controllable than that of those whose propensity is for persons of the opposite sex' (Home Office/Scottish Home Department, 1957: para. 32). In other words, even though homosexual inclination or propensity is not a matter of individual choice, homosexual behaviour is. And, to the extent that behaviour is a matter of choice, so too is it, in principle at least, the province of the law.

In the 1950s and 1960s much debate took place over the proper legal attitude towards the so-called 'victimless crimes': homosexuality, prostitution, drug use, etc. This debate took place in the light of the re-examination of the role of law brought about by the Second World War and the memories of Nazism, though it drew on ideas from much earlier, particularly the liberal principles of John Stuart Mill. The debate was grounded in the distinction between positive and negative freedom as set out by Berlin. A person's freedom to do such-and-such often impinged upon another person's freedom not to have such-and-such done to her/him. As one commentator noted: your freedom to swing your fist in the air stops in close proximity to my nose. The role of law in this case was to balance the positive and negative freedoms. Thus Wolfenden was concerned with creating or allowing homosexual men a freedom to have sex with each other, while seeking '. . . to preserve public order and decency, to protect the citizen from what is offensive or injurious, and to provide sufficient safeguards against exploitation and corruption of others, especially those that are especially vulnerable, because they are young, weak in body or mind, inexperienced or in a state of special physical or economic dependence' (Home Office/Scottish Home Department, 1957: para. 13). This they did by invoking the principle of consent and the idea of privacy (see paras. 63–4). By removing the blanket condemnation of homosexual activity that characterised the earlier law, the Wolfenden proposals certainly provided some degree of liberalisation. But the cost of this was a strict confinement of such behaviour behind closed doors.

The intricate balancing act required of Wolfenden is nowhere more obvious than in the question of the age of consent. As we have seen above, the emergent view was that many people had a degree of homosexual propensity. It seemed axiomatic to the Committee that while allowing the 'doomed' to indulge in homosexual sex, everything should be done to discourage others from trying it. In paragraphs 68–75 the Committee engages in a tortuous discussion of the recommended age of consent. In the end the decision is made to recommend 21, rather than 16, for which, on a dispassionate reading, the arguments appear far more convincing. The reasons for preferring an older age depend on the ideas noted above that changes in sexual preference and behaviour were possible into the 20s. They therefore opine: 'While there are some grounds for fixing the age as low as sixteen, it is obvious that however "mature" a boy may be as regards physical development or psycho-sexual make-up . . . a boy is incapable, at the age of sixteen of forming a mature judgement about actions that may have the effect of setting him apart from the rest of society' (Home Office/Scottish Home Department, 1957: para. 71). In other words, you might be mature enough to make a decision to have homosexual sex, but if you choose to do so, you are clearly not mature enough to make the decision (QED).

The Wolfenden Report and the Act of 1967 were liberal measures. They sought to allow that which they found offensive a space at the edge of the society they controlled. This was a measure of their magnanimity and grace. The comment by Lord Arran that '[a]ny form of ostentatious behaviour . . . any form of public flaunting, would be utterly distasteful and would, I believe, make the sponsors of this Bill regret that they have done what they have done' (quoted in Jeffrey-Poulter, 1991: 90) was a not terribly subtle reminder that what the Lords had given, the Lords might take away. Homosexuals were to be grateful for what they had been allowed, go away and not frighten the horses.

That the liberal case could, as Weeks suggests, have become irrefutable by 1967 is not due simply to the strength of the argument. It was not simply a rational process of social change. Its success is even more surprising when we consider the series of homosexual scandals in the 1950s and 1960s. Enactment of the Wolfenden proposals needed the Labour Government of 1966–70 with its swinging majority. It needed the mood of technological hyperactivity that the government represented (at least until the sterling crisis of 1967). It also needed the support of a great Home Secretary, Roy Jenkins. But the roots of the liberal victory lie in a longer-term process of social and sexual liberation. It depended on the decline of mass movements and proletarian solidarity and the emergence of individualistic, conscience politics. It needed the decline in deference to authority that the end of the war had accelerated but which society had been working towards over a long period.

Coming of Age and Coming Out

Ten years after the publication of the Wolfenden Report, a Labour Government, following very closely Wolfenden's recommendations, passed the Sexual Offences Act (1967) decriminalising certain, tightly defined homosexual acts, while increasing the penalties available for others. The law which resulted is often inconsistent, usually unclear and always confusing (see Crane, 1981: 65–72). However, in the same way that, since the emergence of AIDS, a generation has grown up knowing nothing other than the need for safer sex, so the passing of the Act allowed a generation to grow up relatively free from the threat of blackmail and legal prosecution which characterised the period until 1967. It would, however, be quite wrong to ascribe to the Act too much influence in the creation of what today we recognise as gay culture. This arises from another historical coincidence: the passing of the 1967 Act and the almost contemporary rise of a worldwide gay liberation movement.

The roots of the gay liberation movements and the social conditions that allowed their success were quite different from those which allowed the liberal measures. The beginning of the gay liberation movement is traditionally dated from the Stonewall Riots of June 1969. During a (routine) raid on the Stonewall, a gay bar in Greenwich Village, New York, a group of streetwise drag queens resisted police and sparked a riot which lasted for three days (see Marotta, 1981; Humphreys, 1972). While this event provides a convenient focus for gay pride (and celebrations are held annually in many cities in the USA and Europe on the last Saturday of June to commemorate the event), it is important not to ascribe to the Stonewall Riots more influence than they had at the time. They are better regarded as a watershed in, not the inception of, a movement.

The events at the Stonewall Inn were neither unprecedented nor unique. There was a tradition of resistance to police raids on gay bars both in New York and in San Francisco. The influence of Stonewall was its ignition of a particular part of New York at a particular time in history. Already the home to the 'counter-culture', the Village provided a fertile mixture of radical politics, theoretical insight and physical determination which allowed the resistance to go beyond the immediate to the general.

The crucial shift in consciousness that enabled the riots and the movement is the shift from acceptance of homosexuality as an unfortunate disability to the celebration of being gay as a potentially fulfilling, life-enhancing experience, with no more nor less intrinsic moral worth than heterosexuality. Many American historians date the change to a pamphlet by Frank Kameny, a civil servant dismissed by the American government for his homosexuality, entitled 'Gay Is Good' (1969). The change deliberately echoed the contemporary move from black civil rights to black power as encapsulated in the slogan 'Black is beautiful'.

As we have indicated earlier, gay pride finds historical pre-echoes at least as far back as the late nineteenth century, but, like so-called second wave feminism in the same period, gay liberation seemed to be an idea whose time had come as the explosive spread of ideas and their ready acceptance fuelled an efflorescence into what we now recognise as the gay community. However diverse that community is or becomes, whatever the fundamental disagreements it fosters, the insight remains: the assertion of the authentic and unassailable dignity of gay existence.

The ideas of American gay liberation were brought back to Britain in 1970 by Aubrey Walter and Bob Mellors. They organised a series of meetings, first at the London School of Economics. The gay liberation movement, as it developed, created a politics of identity, central to which was the adoption of 'gay' to replace the term 'homosexual'. This marked not only the rejection of the medical and positivist discourse of sickness, pathology and cure that had bedeviled so many lives, but also emphasised the fact that gay men were self-created: they forged for themselves in this period not only an identity, but a community and a sense of self-worth on a scale that is arguably unique in history. As Foucault has commented, 'Gays have taken an important, interesting step: they define their problems differently by trying to create a culture that makes sense only in relation to a sexual experience and a type of relation that is their own. [They take] the pleasure of sexual relations away from the area of sexual norms and its categories and in so doing [make] the pleasure the crystallising point of a new culture' (Barbadette, 1982: 39). Crucial and central to its program was the need to come out — as a process of individual growth and community solidarity. Consciousness raising and 'happenings' facilitated this pattern. Weeks (1977: 190) has written:

> The GLF recognised three external types of oppression: persecution (largely legal but also physical in the phenomenon of 'queer-bashing'); discrimination (in jobs, in housing, in cases involving child custody, in meetings, in displaying signs of affection in public); and thirdly, 'liberal tolerance'. . . . Increasingly, this supercilious 'acceptance' came from the media, the psychiatric and medical professions — but in its generosity it reaffirmed its superiority. [2] . . . there was a fourth, more dangerous form of oppression — self oppression, the internalisation of guilt, of self-hatred, of the values of the oppressors. (Weeks, 1977: 190)

Weeks (1977: 191ff.) goes on to identify three basic projects of the Gay Liberation Front (GLF) as 'coming out', 'coming together' and 'thirdly and centrally, the identification of the roots of oppression in the concept of sexism.' Coming out consisted of three parts: to oneself, to other 'homosexuals' (sic) and to other, straight people. GLF also 'challenged the exploitativeness of the traditional gay commercial scene'. In this and in its other methods of drawing attention to its demands, it pre-dates by twenty years the 'radical queers' of the 1990s. (Gay liberation was a euphoric experience for those who encountered it in the early 1970s. This comes over in the style of the writing. Compare Weeks' style in his chapter on GLF with that on earlier periods of British history, and a breathlessness born of excitement is still discernible.)

Born of the New Left, the GLF was a primarily middle-class, white and intellectual movement. Weeks characterises the supporters of GLF as having '. . . a high proportion of artists, drop-outs, social security claimants and the young . . . — that is those who had least to lose by being defiantly open. But it also had a high percentage of new professional people, of student teachers and sociologists (who provided much of the drafting and linguistic skills)' (Weeks, 1977: 190–1); although one has to say that the notion of sociologists providing linguistic skills does not fill one with confidence.

The rejection of medical and scientific objectification and the demands to explore the authentic experience of being gay led to a deep and abiding distrust of the methods of the natural sciences in general and the positivist project in particular. The basic texts of the new movement (which must include Altman, 1971; Plummer, 1975; Weeks, 1977; Tripp, 1975) were overtly or implicitly hostile to scientific method, enquiry and modes of explanation. It is this hostility which underpins the ambivalence of the alliance forced between the movement and the medical profession by the threat of AIDS.

The GLF as a coherent movement foundered on questions of organisation and direction. Disagreements emerged between those who looked for a diverse movement, without organisation, and those who wished to move towards more structure of membership and hierarchy; between those who saw the main focus as gay issues and those who sought a common cause with feminists. But in many ways GLF ended because its job was done. As Jeffrey Weeks says, 'The essence of GLF was to change consciousness. But once it had begun to change it . . . it seemed less necessary to build the sort of radical movement that GLF claimed was necessary to carry it through. GLF's revolutionary rhetoric masked . . . reformist aims, ones which could be attained within the framework of liberal bourgeois society' (Weeks, 1977: 205).

Decline or Diversity?

From the mid-1970s, however, organised gay politics went into what appeared at the time to be a terminal decline. Petty issues and utopian dreams obsessed the few and distanced the many, who preferred to dance than to demonstrate. The challenge of the GLF to the commercial scene was clearly a signal failure. It is worth distinguishing three aspects of this process.

Radical Politics

Gay liberation was born of the New Left, with its humane Marxist agenda of liberating the individual from the constricting toils of capitalism. In Britain the early movement was, as the comments from Weeks indicate, heavily influenced by continental philosophy. As the movement grew, diversified and established itself, certain of the intellectual fathers became embroiled in the sinuous and intellectually strenuous debates between the various analyses of structuralism, post-structuralism, deconstructionism and post-modernism. There can be little doubt that these debates excited few of the millions of gay men who, paradoxically, owed their liberated outlook to an intellectual movement transformed into a mass movement.

Early gay liberation made a trenchant and radical case that the oppression of lesbians and gay men was inextricably linked to gender oppression. This link between the agenda of the gay movement and feminism, despite its theoretical strength, did not survive in practical politics for very long, and the history of the movement in the late 1970s was one of rifts and bitter debates on the issue of gender differences, particularly on the links between the needs of lesbians and those of gay men. The re-fusion of what became a myriad of groups did not emerge until the end of the 1980s.

Political Organisation

Over the past twenty years the American gay liberation movement has become assimilated to the American political system to the extent that a ritual obeisance to lesbian and gay concerns forms an obligatory part of the speech of any Democratic Presidential aspirant. In Britain this has not happened and there are, broadly speaking, two reasons for this. On the one hand, the diversity of political organisation in the United States, where political success often depends on the building of coalitions between minorities, provides a fertile ground for an organised gay and lesbian voice — and so it has proved. On the other hand, the monolithic, centralised power structures of British macro-politics are far less suited to such influences. The two parties with their persistent class agendas and firm central control do not generally encourage diverse voices.

Nevertheless, during the late 1970s and early 1980s a significant and partially successful attempt to give practical expression to lesbian and gay concerns was made at the level of local politics. During the late 1970s many gay men and lesbians joined local Labour parties, and in the early 1980s a number of left-wing councils emerged in the metropolitan cities, particularly London and Manchester. These councils were dominated by a New Left, which was urban, middle-class and radical. Immediately termed the 'loony left' by the reactionary press, they established a radical agenda which looked to the needs of a 'rainbow coalition' of the dispossessed: the poor, women, black people, lesbians and gays. In this way they sought to build a majority of minorities on the American model. This majority would replace the declining working-class vote in the large cities, and the agenda would put into practice some of the ideas of the New Left. Council committees which addressed the needs of these constituencies emerged, and in some places real action was taken to improve the lot of gay men and lesbians. This agenda became the focus of vituperative hostility of the gutter press and the tory 'qualities'. Funding of gay — or particularly lesbian — organisations was used, without further justification, to show the 'looniness' of the councils. The metropolitan councils were eventually abolished by the Tory Government in the late 1980s despite popular opposition.

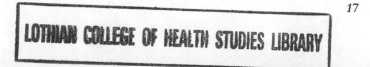

The Growth of Diversity

Perhaps the most important development of the 1970s was the growth of the gay community in Britain. From its small beginnings, groups of women and men began to form in cities and towns throughout the country. What they created was an infrastructure, a set of spaces within which gay lives could be lived. These consisted of social groups and commercial venues, special interest meetings and 'gay nights' at run-down pubs. Most important were the articulating structures, those helplines, switchboards and advice lines which put people in touch with one another and provided support to individuals in the process of coming out. Central to this was the development of a gay press. In the late 1970s some of the large cities began to create gay centres — actual buildings to foster and house the vibrant diversity of gay life.

Today a glance at the listings page of a gay newspaper shows groups encyclopedic in their range and dazzling in their diversity. It is, perhaps, easy to scoff at gay train spotters, but the proliferation of the groups shows that the need to be gay is not something that is restricted to the bedroom, the cruising ground or the disco, and individuals refuse to confine their gay existences within these bounds. Most important, though, is the emergence of a generation of young gay men and lesbians for whom coming out, while individually difficult, was a much more ordinary process than for their older brother and sisters, and a generation of young people in general for whom homosexuality was far less an issue than for many older people.

When the first decade of gay liberation was considered in 1980, a certain sense of pride was justified. A community had emerged from nothing. Great strides had been made in establishing the infrastructure of a gay community. A generation of lesbians and gay men was beginning to carve out careers in a wide range of professions and trades. New challenges were emerging, with the election of the Tories in 1979, and old hostilities remained: in public opinion, in violence, in discrimination. Public figures still risked their careers if they came out, or were dragged out by the tabloid press. Overall, there was a lack of common purpose in the community, as it strove towards a realistic and realisable political agenda. But the sense that gay liberation was irreversible was common, if not universal. The arguments were over future objectives, not the defence of current gains. In 1980 we looked forward to another decade of change and progress.

> One of the problems we have is the desire to see the gay movement as a political party, wanting to initiate national campaigns and organisations and then feeling we have failed when this does not succeed. We should recognise that the gay movement as it has evolved until now takes on a multitude of forms rather than being a coherent organisation with agreed goals. . . . The unifying element in this diversity is the validation of the gay experience and identity and the development of the gay community. . . . It is only through activities at all levels such as these that a stronger and more widely based community can be built and from this have the power to challenge the oppression we face as gays. (Birch, 1980: 92)

And then there was AIDS.

Notes

1 There is a voluminous literature on the distinction between the homosexual and the invert and, indeed, other labels which will not detain us here.

2 It is sobering to see the same mechanisms of oppression as the focus of the new agitators of the 1990s. However great the impact of gay liberation, and it should be neither underestimated nor scoffed at, the institutionalisation of heterosexism is resilient and long-lived.

3 A Brief History of HIV Education

But we dream we are rooted in earth — Dust!
Flesh falls within sight of us, we, though our flower the same,
Wave with the meadow, forget that there must
The sour scythe cringe, and the blear share come.
(Hopkins, 779)

There is not one history of AIDS. Just as we each have our own personal history of acquaintance with HIV, so each group has its own diary of significant events, its own gallery of hero(in)es and hate figures, its own political agenda. The events around which medical histories (e.g., Siegal and Siegal, 1983; Cahill, 1983, especially Part 1; Connor and Kingman, 1988) are woven record the growth of expert, medical knowledge. Its heroes — mostly masculine — are the scientists, and its agenda is medical control of the epidemic. State histories (e.g., Nichols, 1989; Strong and Berridge, 1990) are punctuated by the moves of governments. They have few individual heroes, but are populated by public institutions and the pronouncements of public figures. Their agenda, disguised in academic 'objectivity', is the rationalisation of AIDS: its reduction to an exercise in liberal policy-making. The gay communities have, as a group, the longest history of engagement with the problems of HIV and — consequently or contingently — the most fragmented view of the history of the epidemic (see, for example, Shilts, 1987; Crimp, 1989; Watney, 1987).

Thus it can be seen that the work of historians is not value free. It does not consist simply of recording faithfully an agreed sequence of events, but is a necessarily partial selection, interpretation and presentation of them. It is a resource of privilege and an exercise of power. The privilege of writing history is not confined to those who call themselves historians but, more generally, to the eloquent, the educated and, most potently, those with positions within the academy or other institutions validated by the state. The most potent exercise of power in the writing of history is the process of exclusion: of writing out. Simply not to mention an individual or a group or a social movement is the most certain form of exclusion, which has served to perpetuate the powerlessness of many groups. Over the last quarter-century or so this exclusion has been challenged by scholars from within the historically disadvantaged (overlapping) groups: black people, women, lesbians and gay men.

The process of writing out of history continues before our very eyes, even today. Over the last decade the history of the lesbian and gay movement, and of the men and women who comprise it, has been profoundly shaken by HIV and AIDS. Our communal memory recalls the fight to formulate a set of responses to AIDS in the early years of the epidemic, from 1981. At a time when governments and the mass of the medical profession saw AIDS as unimportant and the lives and deaths of those with the syndrome as beneath notice and contempt, the gay communities of North America and Europe formulated the notion of safer sex, created the means to support people living with HIV, raised the funds to provide these services and to carry out vital basic research, chivvied medical services into taking the problem seriously and agitated for state responses to a global catastrophe in the making. Governments began to take notice and action in about 1986. Since then, some gay men and lesbians have become the mainstay of the AIDS industry; the models of support and care established in the early years have been more widely promulgated; and the contribution of the communities is being systematically written from the records.

The histories of AIDS begin in 1986 with government response. The time of struggle before that date is ignored. The response to AIDS is assimilated to an establishment history, to the triumphalist discourse of modern medicine and the courage and sacrifice of those who died fighting the ravages of their bodies. The sick, sullen and savage prejudice of their societies is simply elided. We owe it to their memory, to our present anger and grief at the continuing epidemic and our pride in facing it and, most importantly, to the future generations of gay men and lesbians to resist this act of exclusion, to record our sorrow, our anger and our pride; to document our own history; and to challenge the enormous condescension of those who, through ignorance, malice or simple stupidity, will deny us our memory and our history.

A History

The aim of this chapter is modest: to provide a brief outline of some of the salient events and features of the epidemic in Britain as it impinged on and was lived by gay men. It is generally agreed that the history of responses to AIDS in the UK should be considered as falling into two periods: from 1981 to 1986 and from 1986 to the present (1993). While other writers may subdivide these periods, (Weeks, 1989; Strong and Berridge, 1990; Berridge, 1992; Freeman, 1992), the importance of 1986, both in the UK and in most of northern Europe (Pollak, 1992), is that it marked the emergence of relatively large-scale state responses.

The peculiar potency of AIDS as a social phenomenon and the main basis of its claim to be, as Sontag (1988) has suggested, 'the disease of the age' lies not only in the emergence of the first major, life-threatening epidemic in the West for some decades, but also its dramatisation and exacerbation of existing lines of social conflict. The history of AIDS plays itself out along and within attempts by the economically liberal and morally conservative national governments of the 1980s to exploit the epidemics to their own advantage, aided, in the UK particularly, by some of the world's most irresponsible and bigoted newspapers. The history of AIDS must be read, therefore, with reference to the long-established, but rapidly accelerating heterosexism of the press, the assault in Britain of the Thatcher

Government on the National Health Service and other public services, the systematic impoverishment of the already poor at the cynical expense of the already very wealthy and the promulgation of a myopic and morally bankrupt social agenda, all promoted under the disarming banner of 'traditional family values'. It is from within this matrix that the pattern of response emerged, and it is within this context that its range, content, perspective and scale are to be understood.

Nineteen Eighty-Two

The first British deaths as a result of what became known as AIDS were notified to the Centre for Disease Surveillance and Control (CDSC) in 1982 following reports of a new syndrome of symptoms in the USA in 1981. Brief articles began to appear in the gay press, but as a report of events in the USA, rather than with any sense of urgency. Indeed, in early 1983 the respected but pseudonymous Dr Ray Hamble, medical 'agony uncle' to one of the largest groups of gay publications, wrote in answer to a reader's 'letter':

> Dear John, AIDS . . . is probably caused by an unidentified virus which is spreading amongst the homosexual community in the USA and to a very much lesser extent in other countries . . . if there is a virus we don't know how it spreads. AIDS is most common in promiscuous gays with frequent changes of partner. A lot more research is needed, for instance into the particular kinds of sexual technique most commonly associated with the disease. On the bright side there have been VERY FEW cases in Britain and Europe and several so-called cases have proved not to be so. At the most this side of the Atlantic we are talking about handfuls of patients and we need to cut the panic and get our perspectives right. . . . AIDS, even in the USA is like a drop in the ocean [compared to deaths by traffic accidents and smoking]. It is increasing and, of course it is worrying but some of the letters I am receiving on the subject are quite irrational. Short of total abstinence from sexual activity there isn't much advice I can give other than an appeal to keep things in proportion.

While in retrospect this advice appears complacent, two points are worth noting. First, the reference to numbers of letters shows that there was a recognition of a burgeoning problem 'out there' in the community. Second, compared to coverage in the non-gay press, this was informative coverage. For brevity, we have omitted a large section which describes accurately the nosology of the syndrome. This pattern of presenting information in popular publications remains a feature of gay response for some years.

The most fruitful of the reactions in 1982 turned out to be the founding of the Terrence Higgins Trust (THT), named for the first man to die from an AIDS-related illness in Britain and set up by a group of his friends. Prominent among them was Tony Whitehead, who was to become the first chair of THT and one of the most influential figures in British AIDS policy for many years. His subsequent low profile does not diminish the immense debt of gratitude that everyone affected by AIDS in the country owes to him, and does not excuse the conspicuous lack of public recognition for his contributions.

Nineteen Eighty-Three

The founding of the THT was marked by the first conference on AIDS in the UK at the South Bank Polytechnic, an event facilitated by London Lesbian and Gay Switchboard (LLGS) and supported financially by the Greater London Council (GLC) and the then Health Education Council (HEC). The early aims of THT were the collection and dissemination of information about AIDS, the provision of support to people who became ill, particularly through the 'buddying' system, political lobbying and fundraising. Modelled in many respects on the Gay Men's Health Crisis (GMHC) of New York, the THT was from the first organised to enable a diversity of contributions. In this it was able to build on community practice, organising itself in a way familiar to those who knew gay politics of the 1970s. It was able to call on the expertise of many professional gay men, notably but not exclusively gay medics. By harnessing professional competence, community spirit and a great deal of energy, THT was able to establish itself as an authoritative voice in AIDS policy. In the same year the first information leaflet was prepared by the Gay Medical Association (GMA). Although in retrospect its advice was confused and misguided, it may well have had a considerable impact had it not been seized by the Metropolitan Police as an allegedly obscene publication (reported in *The Guardian*, 5 November 1985).

By the middle of 1983 THT had organised several fundraisers and though the response was not overwhelming, sufficient monies were raised to launch the first major health education initiatives. This involved the reprinting and widespread distribution of a GMHC leaflet which promoted the idea that 'the disease' was caused by a sexually transmitted agent. Leafleting activity started in late 1983 and, with a reorganization of THT, progressed on a grand scale in 1984. Leaflets were left in places where they might be picked up rather than presented with opportunity for face-to-face discussion. They focused on biomedical information but their impact was diminished by the jargon used and their rather conservative stance.

In this period the major impact on the gay population was probably made not by the gay press or by the THT but by the mass media and national television. Early in 1983 the first national television documentary was made by the Horizon team for the BBC and called 'Killer in the Village'. This attempt at serious television coverage presented the available facts systematically and seriously, and although projections of the rate of spread were, in retrospect, alarmist, this probably served to heighten the program's impact.

In August 1983 a young boy in Brighton was the victim of a serious and particularly vicious sexual assault by two men, who were never arrested (Watney, 1987: 82). The event led to wide and 'outraged' press coverage, with all the hallmarks of a moral panic (Cohen, 1980). In the context of the burgeoning presentation of AIDS as the gay plague, the anti-gay virulence of the press coverage led many to fear, not without reason, widespread anti-gay violence and, with the re-election of the Thatcher Government with a swinging majority in June, legislative restrictions on gay lifestyles.

It would be wrong to suggest that only gay men reacted to the threat posed by this new epidemic in 1983. Some medical specialists identified the probability that AIDS would become a problem in Britain. In 1983 the Medical Research Council (MRC) established a working party on AIDS (Scramm Evans, 1990: 222), but it was notable that many of those involved, the great and the good of the medical establishment, were not those best informed about the epidemic, nor were they drawn from particularly appropriate medical specialities (see Berridge and Strong, 1990: 237ff.). An important exception was Michael Adler, the first (and at that time the only) professor of genito-urinary (GU) medicine in Britain. Throughout the epidemic his was an important role providing an authoritative medical — and thus acceptable — voice. The role of Adler's clinic at the Middlesex Hospital in London and the (then) Praed Street Clinic at St Mary's Hospital in the early years was critical. As two GU clinics historically popular with gay men, they were almost inevitably at the forefront of AIDS awareness. Both Adler and Dr Tony Pinching of St Mary's played high profile roles for many years — and with considerable credit.

Nineteen Eighty-Four

From 1984 onwards the THT became increasingly well established, setting up its telephone helpline in February (Scramm Evans, 1990: 222), providing services not only for gay men in London but diversifying to include injecting drug users, sex workers and others. It increasingly acted as a model and a resource centre for other agencies which were being set up in cities around the country (Freeman, 1992: 60). New ranges of leaflets were developed and more effectively distributed. Better links were established with the media and other agencies, and a variety of public meetings generated wider interest and involvement in THT and its activities.

Concurrently a few gay men managed to get the issue on the agenda of a few health and local authorities who then began developing their own initiatives (Cotton and Kumari, 1990). These responses were largely reactive, arising either in relation to the health care or social service needs of people with AIDS, or to anxiety, even panic among employees. Few sustained health promotion activities took place in these settings, and the responses of employing authorities and trade unions were often ambivalent (Robertson, 1988).

Capital Gay, a free London-based paper established in 1981, realising that 'splash' headlines might frighten and alienate, chose to run small news items and from July 1984 to June 1986 a weekly column called 'Meldrum on AIDS' appeared (named after its author). This column, rather than force any specific health promotion message, aimed to remind gay men that HIV/AIDS issues had to be addressed. By late 1984 Capital Gay had become the centre for much of the AIDS-related debate. In the early period Capital Gay's contribution to health promotion for gay and bisexual males in London was particularly significant: they supported THT vigorously and provided a forum for rational debate and up-to-date information.

On the medical front the virus that became known as HIV, having been isolated in 1983, was publicly announced to be the cause of AIDS in April 1984 (Altman, 1986: 51; Connor and Kingman, 1988: 30ff.). The discovery of the virus confirmed the growing conviction that the causative agent of AIDS was blood-borne, rather than the effect of immune overload. It is important to note, however, that the need for and the publicising of safer sex among gay men began before this medical watershed (Altman, 1986: 146). It is also notable that the discovery of the virus did not lead overnight to agreement on the nature of safe(r) sex. Many early gay initiatives focused on promiscuity, the need to extol monogamy and to 'know' your partner.

Nineteen Eighty-Five

During 1985 the growing epidemic resulted in a spate of press coverage, beginning with the death of prison chaplain Greg Richards at Chelmsford in January (Berridge, 1992: 16; Vass, 1986: 30; Scramm Evans, 1990: 222; Wellings, 1988: 86), reporting of cleaners threatening to boycott a gay theatre group in February (Watney, 1987: 39) and culminating in the furore over the death of Rock Hudson in the middle of the year (Watney, 1987: 81; Berridge, 1992: 16). In October there was the tragic farce of the mad vicar who threatened to shoot his son should he 'have AIDS' (Watney, 1987: 95), an extreme but not isolated example of Christian charity in response to a real and growing human tragedy.

There can be little doubt that the predominant mood of press coverage at this time was anti-gay, concentrating on the threat posed by the gay plague to innocent victims. Although the grosser references came from the tabloid press, the 'qualities' also saw the epidemic as a way to further the agenda of the New Right. In March the extreme right-wing lobbyist, Digby Anderson, published a diatribe in *The Daily Telegraph* calling for more, rather than less, moral panic and a return to 'traditional moral values' (Watney, 1987: 45). It is clear that press coverage of AIDS ranged from the deeply offensive through the reactionary right-wing to liberal condescension. The gay man in search of information on AIDS could choose the frightening howls of *The Sun* for revenge on 'AIDS carriers', or the chilling calls of Digby Anderson and his squalid ilk for traditional moral values such as detention camps and tattooing, or the simplistic and complacent 'advice' of commentators such as Brian Walden ('stick to one partner and . . . avoid oral and anal sex completely', quoted in Watney, 1987: 102). Alternatively they could follow similar debates in the gay press, though even there the level of fear and consequent recriminations was high and the amount of contradictory information substantial.

It therefore seems quite redundant for Berridge (1992: 22–3) to state that '[t]he furore over "gay plague" representations has tended to overlook their complete lack of policy impact.' That government policy directly focused on AIDS has not entirely followed the line suggested by the intellectual stormtroopers of the right is largely due to the influence of the civil servants in the Department of Health and elsewhere who managed, sometimes obliquely, to impose on their political superiors a more liberal set of responses. It is also due to the sustained critique of the emergent agenda carried out by gay intellectuals, notable amongst them Simon Watney. Berridge completely fails to understand the real and deep fear of many gay men at the time that AIDS would provide the proximate cause of a recriminalisation of homosexual behaviour, something that came a step closer with the introduction of Clause 28 (later Section 28 of the 1988 Local Government Act). She also ignores the fact that government policy only grudgingly acknowledges the existence of a gay epidemic, the lack of funding for health promotion work with gay men and the increasing numbers of attacks on gay men, all of which rely to a greater or lesser extent on the idea that the gay man is at best a second-class citizen, at worst an excrescence to be ripped from the body politic. While the 'gay plague' coverage did not begin this process of vilification and violence, it contributed to the pervasive linkage in the minds of many people between gay men and AIDS: a linkage which is severely detrimental to all concerned.

These events ran in parallel with a series of continuing attacks on the gay community's main articulating institutions. In August the London bookshop Gay's the Word was raided by the police and a number of books, including works by Genet, Hemingway and Sartre, were removed; in October the respected *Gay Times* was prosecuted for sending obscene materials through the post (Watney, 1987: 17, 59). It was not mere paranoia for some people to see in this series of events a concerted effort to disable the gay community, to test the water for more repressive measures. Moreover, the events took place against a background of the concerted attack by the government on all areas of public spending. During 1985 rumours began to circulate that the Public Health Laboratory Service (PHLS) was to be closed or privatised, a move that eventually came to naught. Health Service spending was a prime focus for cuts, and it was far from clear where the 'Thatcherite revolution' was going to end. All that was clear was that it was moving in some very unpleasant directions.

On the positive side, 1985 saw some, albeit hesitant and belated steps by the state to acknowledge the existence of AIDS as a social or public health problem (the terms are used deliberately: it remains far from clear whether the 'problem' is HIV/AIDS or the people who were infecting others). While widespread public concern about AIDS was potentially very embarrassing for the government, Mrs Thatcher and her Cabinet had steadfastly refused to set their ideological stamp on the issue, allegedly because of the Prime Minister's avowed distaste for the entire area. As a result, Donald Acheson, the Chief Medical Officer at the Department of Health and Social Security (DHSS as it then was), had been forced to keep himself well informed about the issue since 1983, and in February he set up an expert advisory group on AIDS (EAGA). However, the government's main action in 1985 was the implementation of a £4 million screening program which aimed to secure the safety of the blood supply. Later in the year the first grant of £35,000 was made to THT; and in December the AIDS Unit was set up within the DHSS to coordinate policy formation and implementation.

Government response at this time, despite the rhetoric of the New Right, was generally in the tradition of public health medicine — a speciality which in the UK has never had high prestige. The pervasive view among policy-makers at the time seems to have been that this was a short-term, medical problem, a viewpoint encouraged by the medics. In June Professor Adler returned from the International Conference on AIDS at Atlanta to say that the vaccine was five years away. This confidence that the cavalry, in the guise of the medical establishment, would arrive in the nick of time was combined with a degree of complacency about the pattern of spread. There is no doubt that the problem was seen as less urgent because it was gay men and 'junkies' who were affected. Indeed, an early response to the problem was to reach for the oldest public health measure in the book: the *cordon sanitaire*. A well attested anecdote relates how the policy of preventing spread of the virus by stopping gay men travelling to London was seriously mooted and (admittedly briefly) discussed at the EAGA.

Nineteen Eighty-Six

During 1986 the pace of response quickened. AIDS became a media 'concern' and there was a spate of television programs, mainly documentaries and discussion programs but also some dramas (Watney, 1987: 98ff.). Television coverage had begun to gather pace with Hudson's death in mid-1985 and was to reach a peak in AIDS Week in early 1987. The voice of television in the epidemic is rather less shrill than that of the press, but still imbued with an aura of liberal condescension. The preoccupation of both documentary and current affairs program formats with the authoritative voice — the calm presentation of information and opinion by an authoritative, often invisible, usually male voice — meant that events are filtered through the preconceptions of the predominantly liberal, exclusively heterosexual — at least putatively — and busy presenters. Thus program-makers controlled the agenda by choosing the experts who were allowed to give their views on the questions they deemed important. In this way ownership of the epidemic was claimed by the establishment who dictated the agenda as medical and public health oriented. By contrast, the community-based initiatives of the gay community were seldom mentioned. Inasmuch as gay men were mentioned, their responses were presented as individual, rather than communal (Alcorn, 1988: 75ff.).

The anti-gay attacks from the right continued, given added impetus by the introduction into one of the country's most popular television soap operas, 'Eastenders', of two gay characters, Colin and his boyfriend Barry. There was a predictable furore (Watney, 1987: 87, 121).

The dominant theme of this burgeoning coverage was the inevitability of a heterosexual epidemic. The assertion that AIDS was a problem that would soon affect every family in the country placed the THT in a dilemma. On the one hand, it was clear that gay men were disproportionately affected by the epidemic and, having established and funded response for a number of years, were in need of substantial support. On the other hand, it was clear that the amount of government funding that would be available for gay initiatives was severely limited. The THT therefore acquiesced in presenting AIDS as everybody's problem (Scramm Evans, 1990: 229; Watney, 1987: 29; Fitzpatrick and Milligan, 1987). Whether, in retrospect, this was a pragmatic strategy or an abdication of responsibility remains a matter of heated debate. Certainly, as Schramm Evans (1990: 229) points out in her extremely partial account of the THT in these years: 'The idea of "everyone" being at risk was a powerful weapon against anti-gay prejudice in 1986, and it was the only one that the gay community, such as that was, had with which to protect itself at a time of brutal public attack.' On the other hand, this preoccupation allows and encourages the lack of provision for gay men.

Whatever the motivations and the eventual verdict, THT was awarded a huge increase in grant during 1986, with a rise to £100,000 (Scramm Evans, 1990: 225). Thus began the major problems in the Trust. At the heart of the problem was the change from a voluntary organisation with a committed group of workers, run on a shoestring budget from a tiny room, to a sizeable organisation with paid staff and volunteers based in its own premises and with a substantial budget to be administered. At the same time the upshot of the 'AIDS is everybody's problem' approach was a diversification of aims and objectives that exacerbated existing friction between volunteers and paid staff, between management needs and the voluntary ethos, between women and gay men, between the radicals and the liberals. These disputes culminated in a number of resignations from THT in mid-1987. It was some time before it regained its direction and dynamism; despite its sterling work, the organisation continues to be prey to frequent crises of management. Such disputes highlighted the necessity for a diversity of organisations providing services and care, as well as education and support around issues of HIV/AIDS. Hence support organisations such as Body Positive and Frontliners emerged from within the THT to offer services that the THT could or would not.

Growing media attention and persistent lobbying led at the end of 1986 to a flurry of government activity. The proximate cause was the report published in October by the US Surgeon General, giving authoritative backing to the heterosexual projections and counselling immediate and substantial intervention. That this should come from an arch conservative lent it, in the eyes of the government at least, further credibility. In November a Parliamentary debate was held, and, while there was little light amongst the heat, this signalled the arrival of AIDS on the national, macro-political agenda. Substantial sums were set aside, a Cabinet subcommittee was set up under the improbable chairmanship of William Whitelaw, and preparations made for a massive public awareness campaign. The Secretary of State for Health, Norman Fowler, visited San Francisco and was photographed shaking hands with an 'AIDS victim', a media 'event' that has little intrinsic meaning or worth. Late in 1986 the Department instructed regional health authorities to set up standing action groups on AIDS (Freeman, 1992: 56).

Nineteen Eighty-Seven

The year began with the government's much heralded leaflet drop through the letterboxes of every home in the country, and in February the television networks cooperated in AIDS Week, a sustained series of programs of some variety. There was, despite the worthiness of the cause, a great deal of worry that the government was seeking to turn the television networks into state propaganda outlets (see Berridge, 1992: 23), a move much in line with New Right ideas.

The DHSS campaign was two-fold. It consisted of the leaflet, entitled 'Don't Die of Ignorance', and short films aired during television advertisement time. The leaflet aimed at bringing the 'facts' about AIDS to the attention of 'the public' in an attempt to encourage *individual* changes in behaviour (Richardson, 1990: 169; Homans and Aggleton, 1988: 159). The short films contained a series of phallic images (icebergs, drills, etc.) and a portentous voice-over which intoned, to the strains of the Dies Irae, 'A New Danger is Stalking the Land'. While the films were a delight for those interested in the symbolism of sex and death, they gave no information about modes of transmission, or strategies for risk reduction, and their most prominent effect was to frighten people.

The leaflets, on the other hand, gave information regarding transmission and prevention and may have proved important contact points for gay and bisexual men as they put the addresses and 'phone numbers of LLGS and THT into every home in the land. The overall efficacy of the campaign has been much debated (Sherr, 1990). On the one hand, it is indeed laudable that the government assumed some responsibility in bringing the issue to the attention of the whole population. On the other hand, the exercise resulted in a great deal of anxiety for people who were alerted to this new danger without being given sufficient information to realistically assess their personal risk.

Although the government had expected some people to want further information on the subject, they had assumed that the helpline at the THT and at LLGS would fulfil these needs. However, British Telecom insisted that the volume of calls might put the exchange out of action, thus forcing the Broadcasters Support Services (BSS) to set up a helpline, largely staffed by THT and LLGS volunteers. After its considerable early success this eventually became the National AIDS Helpline (NAH).

AIDS Week was a coordinated package of programs in different formats and aimed at different audiences. Most were worthy discussions, but there was some effort to address the issue in a light-hearted manner. The week was remarkable for what was probably the freest discussion of sex and sexuality seen on British television. Notable by its absence, however, was any sustained or informed discussion on the needs and responses of gay men (see Watney, 1987: 141ff.).

The media blitz and the spate of government interest resulted in the widespread appearance of AIDS on the agenda of local authorities (Cotton and Kumari, 1990: 215). The Department of Education and Science (DES) issued a circular in November on the need for AIDS teaching in schools (Farquhar, 1991), and the House of Commons Select Committee on Social Services, under the irrepressible Renee Short, began a sustained investigation of the issue. At the same time the reorganisation of the NHS (one of many in the 1980s) led to the reformation of the independent Health Education Council (HEC) as the Health Education Authority (HEA), a move presented as giving it greater access to ministers, but in effect ensuring tighter control over its agenda and output. Since the reorganisation, the HEA has been placed in an extremely difficult position, having to satisfy on the one hand a constituency which demands clear, unambiguous discussion of sex and on the other a paymaster for whom any such discussion is distasteful. The moral campaign of the government on behalf of family values gained pace during 1987 with a series of administrative changes which culminated in the introduction of Clause 28 late in the year. On more than one occasion the government impeded the HEA initiatives, at one time pulping an entire print run of an educational pack because of a single statement about homosexuality.

The discomfort of the government in dealing with this issue was underlined by the setting up of the National AIDS Trust (NAT). This was intended to be the main funding and coordinating body for AIDS prevention and information work in the country. It was to be independent of government, and to be a 'partnership', that is funds would be channelled to it from government, charitable donations and from industry. Such arrangements were a fashionable part of the approach to industrial policy favoured by Lord Young and were aimed at reducing public expenditure. The NAT emerged from an earlier body, the UK AIDS Foundation, set up in 1985, which split over different approaches to testing (Freeman, 1992: 61). In retrospect, the appointment of Robert Maxwell to head its fundraising team is, to say the least, ironic, but it is a matter of record that the NAT never generated the level of funds expected and never played the coordinating role originally envisaged. It remains a relatively small, moderately successful body with vague but modest aims and a bureaucratic structure far too complex for its size.

Tony Whitehead (1989: 108) was quite clear about the government's motivation in setting up the NAT: 'The hidden agenda . . . was how the Government could get away with spending as little as possible. [It] wanted to get as much money from the [gay] community as it possibly could. . . . It was also clear that it wanted to keep itself as far away as possible from any closely targeted education towards gay men and drug users.' He argues strongly that the position of THT at the time was a tactical error. By acquiescing in the government's strategy, it allowed the administration to sidestep its responsibilities. By concentrating on the immediate needs of individuals, he argues, the THT and, by extension the gay community, failed to lobby for an effective government response. 'Instead of simply behaving like so many good little Florence Nightingales, developing our own educational and support services within the gay community, we AIDS activists should have fought for such services within the statutory sector' (Whitehead, 1989: 107). Whether such a strategy was feasible at the time remains debateable, and whether it would have been successful is extremely doubtful.

Following the Conservative Government's re-election in June, the reopening of Parliament was marked by the most serious attack on gay men in the decade, the introduction of Clause 28 of the Local Government Bill. The measure, which aimed to prevent local authorities from 'promoting' homosexuality, was proposed by a group of right-wing Conservatives with tacit government approval and based on similar measures being put forward in the USA. It was aimed directly at the so-called 'loony left' councils, some of which had established lesbian and gay committees. However, the very vagueness of its formulation suggested that it was intended less as a legal weapon, to be used in actual cases against councils, than a spoiling measure, a means whereby the reactionary right could justify its opposition to gay or lesbian initiatives. Indeed, the clause has since its passing into law been used to justify a number of such moves by councils and others. The importance of the Clause is not as an effective piece of legislation but a *carte blanche* to oppose policies and moves towards equal rights for gay men and lesbians. The emphasis on the family in Clause 28 and the associated Clause 25 marks the ideological genesis and myopia of its progenitors.

The clause was met with a massive and sustained campaign by lesbians and gay men and many others who saw it as an outrageous measure. When the veteran campaigner, Antony Gray, compared the clause to the Nazi purges of the 1930s in an early meeting, no-one accused him of overreaction or lack of perspective. At the time the feeling that this was the beginning of a sustained attack on the communities was widespread and justified. Not long after the clause was introduced, and just before it was debated in the House, an arson attack on the premises of Capital Gay lent credence to the fear that the main institutions of gay life were being targeted for destruction — and with the open support of many on the right. For example, Mrs (now Dame) Kellett-Bowman (Lancaster, Con) claimed that it was quite right that Capital Gay had been firebombed since it was an evil institution (*Hansard* 124: 65, 15 December 1987).

The reaction to the clause shows, however, that it is meaningful to speak of the gay and lesbian communities. Faced with a real threat, the scale of the response was impressive. It showed that despite the diversity of experience, political outlook and desire, a common cause subsists in the experience of being a 'sexual outlaw'. The anti-Clause 28 campaign was notable for a number of brilliant coups, mostly from the lesbians, abseiling into the House of Lords was certainly a more imaginative approach to campaigning than the protest march, and the disruption of the BBC's flagship 'Six O'clock News' was daring and innovative, even if it did end with the inoffensive Nicholas Witchell sitting on a dyke. Despite the sustained program of resistance, the stranglehold of the press by the right wing ensured that little news percolated through to the 'general public'.

The campaign was ultimately unsuccessful, but it had two positive outcomes, one minor and legislative and one major and with long-term implications. In the first case an amendment was attached to the clause exempting from its ambit any measure which sought to prevent the transmission of HIV. The long-term effect of the campaign was altogether more consequential and significant. The campaign introduced to the politics of sexuality a generation of gay men and lesbians for whom gay liberation was a vague historical event, about which mustachioed middle-aged men in bars waxed lyrical when the melancholic mood was upon them. After a decade of disco dancing and the confident assertion of the right to life, space and sexual choice, the very real threat of recriminalisation and the recognition that gay life could not be taken for granted but had to be fought for and defended against the forces of repression politicised many, predominantly young people.

The campaign around Clause 28 coincided with the formation in New York of the first chapter of ACT-UP, the driving force behind which was Larry Kramer, another of the heroes of AIDS, who was also central in the founding of GMHC in 1981 (Altman, 1986: 84). Dismissive of the increasingly bureaucratic nature of the organisation, and what he regarded as its complacency, Kramer founded an organisation with street cred to engage in activism aimed at the appalling lack of concern he saw in mainstream American politics. ACT-UP's program of imaginative demonstrations, zaps and actions, and its pattern of democratic organisation and radical outlook was the prototype for many new gay political groups, culminating in 'queer politics', a movement which sought, even in its rejection of what it regarded as the middle-aged conservatism of the gay movement and associated white, middle-class exclusionary organisation, to reinvest sexual politics with some of the revolutionary energy that characterised the early gay movement. Dismissive also of the assimilationist position that many gay activists had in their later years adopted, they celebrated the fact of sexual difference and did so by readopting the term 'queer'. By celebrating the fact of sexual outlawry, by highlighting rather than seeking to play down the challenge posed by homosexuality to the society, the movement sought a *rapprochement* between lesbians and gays, between black and white, between all sexual minorities in a program of claiming space. The reintroduction of the term 'queer' led many gay activists to complain that the main achievement of gay liberation — the adoption of a self-preferred term in place of the medicalising or pathologising discourses — was being squandered in a juvenile attempt to shock.

The campaigns around Clause 28 and around AIDS policy had shown that men and women could work together without agreeing on every issue. The replacement of a demand for Leninist organisation, which characterises claims of weakness in the gay movement, with an anarchic energy led some commentators to regard the movement as juvenile and politically naive. Most queers will not have read Marcuse or Millett, but then neither had the majority of people in the gay liberation movement of the 1970s. Those who had been able to build careers in gay politics and in academia are often guilty of writing a history which privileges the intellectual vanguard and downplays the ordinary. Others have been known to bewail the dissipation of the political energy of the early years in disco dancing, while not recognising that, in many ways, that is what it is all about.

Nineteen Eighty-Eight

On the narrow front of AIDS January 1988 saw the London Conference of Ministers with responsibility for AIDS policy. This conference ended with the signing of the London Declaration, which included a commitment that health education 'should take full account of social and cultural patterns, different lifestyles and human and spiritual values' (quoted in Frankenberg, 1989: 22). Watney (1989: 22) has commented on the irony that, at the same time as the British government was signing up to this statement of liberal acceptance, Clause 28 was being debated in Parliament. It is difficult in retrospect to see what effect the conference had on policy in the UK.

In 1988 the Department of Health published the 'Cox Report' (Department of Health/Welsh Office, 1988), which sought to provide an authoritative prediction of the future course of the epidemic. Concentrating on the period to 1992, the report acknowledged that the task was difficult and more akin to haruspication than science. It was concluded (p. 41) that by 1992 there might be a cumulative total of 10,000 to 30,000 cases of AIDS. In fact, the number reported by September 1992 was 6555 (THT, 1992).

There was continuing trouble at the THT, whose problems seemed to increase with its level of grant, which in 1988–89 was £300,000. The HEA ran a series of adverts in the press, which continued the theme that AIDS was a problem for everyone. On the other hand, THT produced a series of posters aimed specifically at gay men with the slogan, 'Keep it up'. This campaign, under the direction of some of the most trenchant critics of the HEA, was singularly anodyne. Their criticism centred on the need for sexually explicit material for gay men — indeed a laudable and necessary aim. It seemed, however, that raunchy images had a tendency to overshadow the message. Gay men, as a group, are more open to full and frank discussion of sexual techniques than most of the population. It is, however, highly dubious to assume that in order to attract the attention of gay men, you have to have pictures of good-looking young men in varying states of undress and in risqué poses. When these images are accompanied by cryptic messages, such as 'Keep it up' or the HEA's 'Choose safer sex', then we may suspect that the erotic cart is being placed a long way in front of the educational horse.

1988 also saw, perhaps inevitably, a resurgence of the campaign by the right wing to see AIDS work as a 'homosexual' conspiracy. By a neat though scurrilous inversion, they took the fact that the burgeoning AIDS industry was mainly staffed by gay men and interpreted this, not as evidence of the expertise of gay men, or their public-spirited commitment to AIDS work, but as evidence of the invisible peril. They saw a group of perverts subverting the health service and promoting gay rights under the guise of health education.

Nineteen Eighty-Nine to Nineteen Ninety-Two

By 1989 it is probably fair to say that AIDS had become normalised within the British health care system, ravaged though this was by the hostility of the government to any form of public expenditure. This was marked by the instruction by the government that all district health authorities should appoint district HIV prevention coordinators (DHPCs) whose task, as their title suggests, was the coordination of health promotion at the local level (Freeman, 1992: 56). At best, DHPCs manage the complex relationships between statutory and voluntary organisations in a given area to provide a streamlined service and many examples of such good practice exist. At worst, the post is combined with other responsibilities and becomes little more than a sinecure. In many cases, however, DHPCs and local groups have created an infrastructure of care in advance of a significant epidemic in that area. There have been reports of agencies 'fighting' over the few PLWAs in a region, all anxious, ready and willing to provide support on a scale that is not yet needed (see Wilson, 1993). This points to one of the paradoxes of the response to AIDS: the self-defeating prevention program. It is a paradox that the more successful a prevention program is, the less justifiable its existence becomes. If fewer and fewer people come forward with HIV infection, the less justification there is in the market-led NHS for resources to be moved in that direction. The paradox is one which affects all prophylactic medicine in the NHS and is, as yet, unresolved.

The short period since 1986 had seen a change in the status of GU medicine from a backwater attracting the committed few and the low-achieving many, to a fertile base for state-of-the-art medicine and plentiful research funds; the creation from nothing of an 'AIDS industry', with its politically acceptable vocabulary and set of attitudes, its centres of excellence and arcane debates; the gradual growth of AIDS wards and HIV clinics around the country, detracting from, but not eradicating, the pre-eminence of the London centres. The same period has also seen AIDS conferences, coordinating groups, journals, spokespersons and deep divisions. The 'AIDS industry' is disproportionately staffed by gay men and lesbians, most of them products of gay liberation and therefore open about their sexuality, even if their professional remits cover other areas. It is this identifiable concentration of perversion within the apparatus of the state that so inflames the frightened and evil fury of the right.

Despite this, it remains a matter of record that most health authorities have not concentrated on programs of health promotion targeted at gay men (King, Rooney and Scott, 1992). This is due largely to the perceived success of indigenous initiatives which by this time had rendered safer sex normative among many sectors of the gay community — as later chapters of this book will show. The dilemma identified by Whitehead (above) had come back to haunt the gay community: having been successful in informing and protecting themselves without state help, the state then absolves itself of any responsibility to maintain those changes or to provide further help or support. Gay men remain outsiders.

The HEA has periodically run media campaigns directed at gay men. These have, until 1992, consisted of large glossy pictures of good-looking young men with minimal text and information. They have been restricted to gay publications and other magazines presumed to have a large gay readership. There have been no campaigns targeted at gay and bisexual men run by the HEA on national media. More positively, the HEA did fund the MESMAC (Men Who Have Sex with Men Action in the Community) project, which is a community development project based in London, Leeds, Leicester and Newcastle. These four sites ran (different) pilot projects aimed at establishing and maintaining safer sexual practices within the (homo)sexual communities in those areas. There is little doubt that the aim of these projects is laudable. As we shall confirm in later chapters, knowledge of safer sex and of unsafe sex is widespread — if not universal — among gay men, yet the practice of safer sex is not. We shall spend some time considering the reasons for this, but the aim of identifying, promulgating and reinforcing safer sex within sexual communities is to be welcomed in that it moves beyond the mere giving of information to the far more intractable problem of putting that knowledge into effective practice.

On the other hand, the project has been criticised for its slow delivery, though this is perhaps unfair, and for its failure to investigate the local needs of the communities it sought to educate and empower. Latterly, local needs assessments have become popular with health authorities. Criticised for their lack of targeted interventions for gay men, many district authorities have seized upon the idea of assessing the need for programs in their areas. While such moves are to be welcomed as beginning to redress the historic avoidance of gay men's needs and issues, such exercises can become the merest tokenism. In the best case, needs assessments should be only the first step in a program. All too often, unfortunately, they are the one and only signal of concern by the authority. It also seems that many such exercises are poorly focused, concentrating on gathering information which is of dubious relevance.

Many of the most trenchant critics of the statutory sector's response to HIV came together in 1992 to form Gay Men Fighting AIDS (GMFA). Their aims are:

> to promote safer sex amongst gay men, to monitor the suitability and appropriateness of services for gay men with HIV or AIDS, and to challenge homophobia both in terms of institutional neglect and active prejudice. It was formed by a group of gay men in an attempt to rectify the imbalance between the small proportion of HIV prevention resources specifically targeted towards gay men and their continued existence as the group most severely affected by the epidemic. (Scott, 1992: X7–8)

The formation of GMFA embodied the growing disenchantment of some of the most vocal among AIDS activists with various aspects of the AIDS industry. Central to those concerns, as the quotation above indicates, is the 'imbalance' between need and resources. To highlight this imbalance, there have been some moves to reintroduce the idea of risk groups. To many, this has been a baffling reversal of the earlier moves which sought to eradicate the usage, except in its strict, technical sense (see below, Chapter 4).

The renewed arguments about the term 'risk group' are misplaced. They are also misguided in diverting debate from the main issue: the relationship of the gay community to society in general. The original case against use of the term 'risk group' was that it made social identities stand for physical processes. Thus it was rightly pointed out that being gay did not make a man susceptible to HIV; rather, his portfolio of risk behaviours did. To the extent that a group of men who did not describe themselves as gay also engaged in, say, anal intercourse, then the term became misleading. The phrase 'men who have sex with men' was coined to describe the epidemiological category of men who were at putative risk. This usage is quite correct, but it is now suggested that the term has come to be used in a way that excludes (rather than incorporates) the gay community. Programs that have been developed under this term have, it is argued, systematically played down the needs of gay in favour of the non-gay identified men (see Dowsett *et al.*, 1992).

What GMFA and others aim to do is to draw attention to the fact that the gay community is disproportionately affected by the ravages of HIV and, most trenchantly, that it serves as an effective mechanism for health promotion. Thereby, they seek to mould together a health and a political agenda, since encouragement of gay community enables and encourages better health, including safer sex. By locating safer sexual practice within a real community context, within wider health care needs, the group seeks to move away from the individual, specific emphasis of earlier approaches, towards the normalisation of HIV within the community.

It is still too soon to evaluate the effectiveness, let alone the success of GMFA. There is much which leads to optimism. Unlike the HEA or the THT, they are not beholden in any way to the government. Unlike ACT-UP, they are committed to positive programs. Unlike most other agencies, they espouse appropriate, that is to say raunchy, sex education materials for gay men and low-level interventions rather than high-profile and vacuous media campaigns. In this they seem more attuned to the current state of the epidemic than most agencies.

Final Thoughts

AIDS is an appalling and continuing tragedy. Despite its scale, so habituated have we become, that the news that a friend of a friend has died often occasions little more than perfunctory sympathy. The direct effects of infection, our own or that of our close friends, remain as searingly apocalyptic as they have ever been, or will ever become. Yet it requires an effort of intellect and will to make the connection between the immediate, real, devastating effects of personal acquaintance and the long-term, complex and often dispiriting agenda for community or national action. The relevance, the appropriateness, the effectiveness of large-scale, long-term, diffuse programs are all called into question by the anger, commitment and absolute facticity of infection. Yet it remains undeniably true that over the last decade there have been some people, and gay men have been numerous and prominent among them, who have harnessed the anger and the concern to create the response to HIV that we have documented, however partially (in both senses of that word) in this chapter.

It is easy, in the aura of anger which the reading of these histories so often engenders, to forget the successes that have punctuated the decade of AIDS. While it would be crass to suggest that HIV had been a general or a net benefit to anyone or any community, it would also be inaccurate to suggest that no good has come of it. There can be little doubt that the epidemic has given the gay community a potent rallying point, that the AIDS industry has increased the visibility of gay men in a number of organisations where they are visible as gay men and that many of the demands of gay libration have been rendered more trenchant by the fact of AIDS. These in no manner outweigh or compensate for the devastation and misery of the epidemic, but the community should be proud while it retains its anger, confident while it keeps its commitment, and forward-looking while it remembers the past.

4 Metaphorical Constructions

Because night is here and the barbarians have not come
Some people arrived from the frontiers
And they said that there were no longer any barbarians.
And now what shall become of us without any barbarians?
Those people were a kind of solution

(C.P. Cavafy)

To many people some of the time and to some people most of the time, the emphasis placed by some activists on politically acceptable terminology must have seemed misplaced. The moves to replace 'AIDS victim' with PWA, then with PWHIV, PLWA, for example, or the furore over the term 'risk group' can appear to be the most fastidious irrelevance. Yet the refusal to accept demeaning terminology and the attempt to assert control over the language of AIDS is one of the most striking features of the history of the epidemic. A recognition of the power of words, an appreciation of the importance of discourse in understanding the problems of AIDS sprang from the history of gay liberation, where, as we have noted in Chapter 2, much attention was focused on the creative power of language, not least in the creation of the term 'gay'.

The concern with terminology is no mere shibboleth, but stems from a conviction that our experience as humans is shaped by language, not simply reflected in it. Discourse analysis, in particular, is concerned with the ways in which the metaphors we employ direct our thoughts and our actions. It is also centrally concerned with the ways in which particular metaphors, particular ways of speaking, empower some groups over others. In Chapter 2 we have reproduced some of the words used by liberal reformers of the 1950s. 'Homosexuals', in their terms, are 'hopeless' cases, 'doomed' to a sad and sorry existence on the 'margins of society'. Gay liberation has largely succeeded in replacing this language with one that speaks of happiness, pride, power and authenticity, yet the condescension of the liberal continues (see Ruse, 1988: *passim*).

A detailed disquisition on the relation of language to thought to action is beyond the scope of this volume, but we note the way that metaphor flourishes around illness (Gilman, 1988). The locus classicus of contemporary analysis is Susan Sontag's influential essay, written in response to her own experience of cancer. Sontag draws out the metaphoric implications of the ways in which we talk about illness and asserts that 'illness is not a metaphor and the most truthful way of regarding illness — and the healthiest way of being ill — is the one most purified of, most resistant to metaphoric thinking' (1978: 3). It is doubtful, however, if such refinement of thought is possible for, as Grover (1989: 152) has pointed out, 'language is itself a metaphor and we can no more "purify" it in discussing disease than in describing a beautiful day or how love makes us feel.' To this extent, therefore, the metaphors which are used in order to understand AIDS and HIV are central to understanding our responses to the epidemic and the patterns of empowerment and disempowerment that these metaphors create in their wake.

The Body and Society

All collectivities of people — nations, cultures, even special interest groups such as train spotters — exist and define themselves in opposition to the rest of the world. Each is defined by its difference and that which separates it from the rest of the world. In the latter part of the nineteenth century, from the patchwork of political allegiances on the continent of Europe slowly emerged a collection of nation states, each determined to assert its difference and its superiority to its neighbours. Under the impetus of this competition a new concern began to define itself, a concern with the health of the nation. It manifests itself in the health fads of the late nineteenth century: nudism, vegetarianism, rational dress; in the chauvinism of national histories; and in the questions of birth control, racial purity and 'public health' which, together, characterised the eugenics movement.

While this concern with national superiority, racial purity and manifest destiny reached its terrible apotheosis in Nazi Germany, all the countries of Europe shared and developed these concerns and central to the nationalist program was the extirpation of the alien, the outsider and the degenerate. Jews and gypsies suffered because of their wilful refusal to confine themselves to national boundaries. Homosexuals of both genders suffered because they represented a failure, a degeneracy, a weakness to be ruthlessly eradicated. As we have argued above, the need to distinguish 'us' from 'them' is a pervasive, maybe a necessary, feature of human interaction. What the nationalist project provided, however, was a particularly powerful source of metaphor, one which has, revived in the age of AIDS, been remarkably insistent and pervasive. It may be summarised thus: 'disease is to body as invasion is to nation.' The metaphor invites us to see:

- the nation as an integrated, interdependent, organic whole, as is the body

The representation of the nation or the tribe or the society as a body is widespread (see Douglas, 1966) and present in such phrases as 'the body politic', 'Britain took *x* to its heart', 'the nation's manhood' — particularly interesting that one, since it equates militarism with virility (see Theweleit, 1989). It lies behind the personification of the nation as Britannia, John Bull, etc. and it ramifies into ideas such as 'the family of nations' and so on.

- threats to the nation in terms of disease

It is not unusual to hear invasions referred to as 'the cancer in our midst'. During the debates over law reform in the 1960s the journalist Monica Furlong referred to the feeling among the reactionary right that 'a moral rot may well have set into our national life.' Otherwise, it was argued that 'respectable millions [of ordinary people] must not be contaminated by a few minions' (quoted in Jeffrey-Poulter, 1991: 73, 77).

- the effects of disease on the body as the effects of invasion

Of particular note in our area of concern is the visualisation of the immune system as the 'defences' of the body. (A popular textbook on the working of the immune system is entitled *The Body at War*). The image of invasion is present in the graphics, beloved of television producers, which portray the immune system as star wars — a battle of abstract shapes in space, rather than a series of immensely complex but infinitesimal chemical reactions.

The identification of what became known as AIDS among homosexually active men in 1981 (Gottlieb *et al.*, 1981) led to an explosion of signification, to a burgeoning complexity of metaphor, an understanding of which is no mere intellectual gymnastic, but central to an understanding of the responses to HIV and AIDS in the 1980s.

The Invasion of the Body

Watney (1989: 20) has distinguished two dominant metaphors in AIDS commentary, which he terms the 'terrorist' and the 'missionary'. The former thrives on ideas of HIV as 'an external invader', whereas in the latter the virus is 'essentially understood as a kind of evil spirit, taking possession of its victims.' Rather than a terrorist, however, surely the unifying metaphor for HIV must be drawn, as Miss Prism might say, from espionage. The figure of the 'sleeping' secret agent, the 'mole', as described by le Carré, describes both the action of the virus within the body and the reactions at national level with uncanny accuracy.

At the somatic level the virus' actions are those of the good mole. Infiltrated to the body through invasive procedures — penile penetration, syringe injection — it insinuates itself into the body's own 'defence system', there to lie dormant for some time before becoming active to turn the body's defences against themselves. 'Unlike previous epidemic diseases, which have usually slipped through the intricate network of the immune system, AIDS destroys the fibre of the system itself' (Siegal and Siegal, 1983: 1). In itself, the image of the subtle virus, the virus as mole, is harmless, and it might be argued that, if, as we have suggested above, metaphoric thought is inevitable, then this metaphor is as good as any other. But this is not so. In a subtle but most insidious way, this metaphoric trope empowers the medical profession and enables a particular set of responses — medical, scientific, expert — at the expense of others — community, cooperative, consolidating.

The invasive agent of altogether unprecedented deviousness requires an adversary of superior subtlety. How many scientists have not seen themselves, if only fleetingly, as the lugubrious, brilliant but immensely reassuring George Smiley. Drawing on a different genre for illumination, Williamson (1989: 71) writes: 'the classic horror film . . . involves a search for specialist forms of knowledge: in most vampire films, a Goodie has at some stage to find an ancient leather bound volume which explains how to put a stake through the heart of a vampire and usefully mentions that demons can't stand garlic or the sign of the cross.' She continues: '. . . we are accustomed to expecting specialist knowledge to allow comprehension, control and ultimately elimination of the threat. Medical knowledge is most frequently seen in this light, as if each problem were a keyhole merely waiting for a particular key.' Scientists involved in understanding the virus become, in *Time*'s phrase, 'Disease Detectives Tracking the Killers' (see Altman, 1986: 17). By casting the virus in the role of intellectual adversary, we are encouraged to look for the solution with the expert, with the specialist and with the medical profession.

The medicalisation of AIDS is buttressed by the triumphalist discourse of modern medicine (see, for example, Siegal and Siegal, 1983: 171–2; Nichols, 1989: 304–9). Advances in surgical and particularly chemical techniques over the last century and the consequent (but sometimes contingent) eradication of diseases have encouraged medics to present themselves as the answer to the problems of AIDS. They are, in their eyes, the ones with the technology who, given the resources, will provide the solution. This belief in the ability of medicine to provide the answers is explicit in the way that a cure or a vaccine is always presented as imminent. In 1985 Professor Adler returned from the Atlanta conference saying that a vaccine was five years away. Reports from the Amsterdam conference of 1992, seven years later, put the discovery of the vaccine five years in the rapidly receding future.

Vast resources have been poured into the search for the solution: a cure, a vaccine; and there is no doubt that great strides have been taken in understanding a remarkably complex and recalcitrant problem, summed up in the words of Brandt: 'At no time in history has so much progress been made on such a complex disease in so short a time' (cited in Plummer, 1988: 25). This phrase has been repeated many times in the first decade of AIDS, with increasing desperation and sounding increasingly hollow as the years pass, for in that decade the most trenchant and successful responses to AIDS came not from the laboratories but from the streets. It is noteworthy in this respect that the patients often had a better grasp of the medical complexities of nosology, diagnosis and regimens of care than the ostensible experts (Horton, 1989: 162ff.).

For the medicalisation of AIDS has never gone unchallenged (Plummer, 1988: 24ff.). The imperatives of the burgeoning epidemic forced gay men into an ironic alliance with the medical profession. The first irony was the partial rapprochement with the very group (medics, natural scientists) from whose baleful control gay liberation had successfully extricated itself in the 1970s (see Chapter 2; Altman, 1986: 50ff.; Plummer, 1988: 26).

Hunt the Homosexual

It is possible to read the writings of Krafft-Ebing and the rest as manuals for the identification of the sexually degenerate. Specifically for the use of medics and jurists, these texts make no secret of their nationalist project:

> The episodes of moral decay [in the history of civilisation] always coincide with the progression of effeminacy, lewdness and luxuriance of the nations. . . . The material and moral ruin of the community is readily brought about by debauchery, adultery and luxury. Greece, the Roman Empire and France under Louis XIV and XV are striking examples of this assertion. In such periods of civic and moral decline the most monstrous excesses of sexual life may be observed. . . . (Krafft-Ebing, 1925: 6)

The need for such manuals of identification arises from the invisibility of the homosexual, more precisely his ability to seem 'normal' in everyday life (to 'pass' in Goffman's (1968) term). The frantic search for the stigmata of the homosexual that Sedgewick (1990) documents is a search for certainty, a search for the undeniable mark of the beast. In the same way that the sexologists list the marks of the homosexual, so authors of fiction describe his or her characteristic behaviour, demeanour and appearance. But this game of 'hunt the homosexual' is not confined to the scientific and the literary. In schools the search for the mark was and no doubt remains a popular pastime.

More potently, and in greater complexity, the metaphor of the invisible peril applies to the reactions of individuals and collectivities of individuals. Like homosexuality, AIDS becomes 'the cancer in our midst', a threat to the national health which calls for the mobilisation of the nation in a fight/battle/war against AIDS, or an attempt to identify and extirpate the 'invisible peril', Altman (1986: 30) has sought to understand reactions to AIDS in the USA with reference to the movie, *The Andromeda Strain*. Perhaps the more appropriate cinematic representation is *Invasion of the Body Snatchers*, itself a straightforward metaphor for the hysterical search for communists in McCarthyite America.

At the heart of this battle at the societal level is the search for that which marks the carrier, for by a simple metonymic shift, the carrier becomes assimilated to the threat itself. As Watney (1989: 19) has written, 'instead of being understood as a group at high risk of contracting HIV, gay men are widely regarded as constituting a high risk to other people.' It is through this process that the person with AIDS becomes the focus not of compassion but of ostracism, fear and loathing. The important notion of the 'high risk group' solidifies the search for the invisible peril by making social identities stand for physical processes.

> By describing the social groups who were first affected by HIV as 'high risk groups', the implication may be incorrectly established that other people are not at risk. With HIV it cannot be sufficiently emphasised that risk comes from what you do, not how you label yourself. There is not intrinsic relation between HIV and any individual or population group. It is therefore advisable to refrain from using the term 'high risk groups'. . . . What should be stressed are risk factors. (Watney, 1989: 185)

This statement remains as true today as it did then.

Most potently, however, the search for the mark of difference is carried out in moral terms, and it is the almost miraculous concordance of the spread of the virus with the preoccupations of the 'moral majority' (Weeks, 1988: 13), enhanced in influence with the election of right-wing governments around 1980, that make the claim of HIV to be the 'disease of the age' a powerful one. Primarily, this difference was sought in non-normative sexuality.

Homosexual practice is condemned primarily for its presumed 'promiscuity' (see below, Chapter 11), for the contention that the rectum is 'not designed for intercourse' (see Watney, 1989: 39) — a bizarre revelation to many of us who had, unwittingly, been using it for that purpose for many years — and in the early 1980s the idea that the homosexual lifestyle, particularly its 'fast-lane' variant, was all too much for the body to stand (Altman, 1986: 35; Alcorn, 1988: 72; Wellings, 1988: 91–2). Not only gay men but also, predictably (by assumption, female), prostitutes become feared vectors of transmission. Gilman (1988: 271) reproduces a notorious cartoon of a group of women, presumably prostitutes, advertising 'Death for Sale', and Williamson (1989: 77) discusses the image of the 'predatory' prostitute. Even in 1992 an unfortunate article by McKeganey (1992) on sex-workers in Scotland had the thoroughly deplorable title 'Hooked on the Killing Game', a preoccupation with the risks posed by these out groups to the presumed pristine majority that is as fundamental to AIDS policy as it is despicable.

Similarly, the distinction between 'guilty' and 'innocent' victims arises from this construction (Plummer, 1988: 33). The guilty are those whose condition is deserved (Wellings, 1988: 87), 'self-inflicted' (Plummer, 1988: 30) or evidence of lack of individual responsibility (Alcorn, 1988: 75). By contrast, the innocent are the children (Gilman, 1988: 268), the female partners of errant males and even the animals used in experiments (Wellings, 1988: 88).

There are consistent attempts also to relocate the origin of the virus and, by implication, blame for AIDS. Gilman (1989: 266) remarks on the deployment of a particularly ancient figure: the sinful city. This figure, with its biblical resonances (see also Brown, 1988: 26–32, 257 *et passim*), derives its contemporary iconic form from Fritz Lang's *Metropolis*. Innumerable television reports and documentaries use footage of the seething, garishly lighted, shadowy world of the gay disco as visual wallpaper to contrast the dark, subterranean, subhuman home of infection with the bright, sunlit uplands of family life.

More widespread are the attempts to locate the origin of the virus in some other region of the world. Thus the Europeans (Altman, 1986: 15) see American tourism as the source of infection, while there is a consistent pedal point of claims that the virus is man-made (Altman, 1986: 10–1; Gilman, 1988: 264). But the Americans are notably uneasy about the construction of AIDS as a disease of (American) civilisation. Thus Shilts' mammoth, indispensable yet tendentious account of American response to HIV (1987) is preoccupied to an altogether unhelpful degree with the identity of Patient Zero, the man who 'brought' the virus to the United States and thus 'started' the epidemic. Early on Haiti, with its convenient associations of despotism and voodoo (Altman, 1986: 39, 71–3; Patton, 1985: 154ff.), figured prominently.

The choice of Africa as the putative source of the virus has a sad inevitability. The displacement of the origin of the virus and, by close linkage, blame from urban America to the 'dark continent' (Altman, 1986: 15; Watney, 1989: 36, 183ff.; Plummer, 1988: 30) enlivens a host of racist discourses, rooted in presumptions of subhumanity and, particularly, hypersexuality (Gilman, 1988: 263) that have influenced immigration policy and allowed some right-wing medics to claim that the heterosexual epidemic is confined to people from Africa. Conversely, in Britain particularly, the assumption within parts of the black communities that homosexuality and AIDS are problems only for white people is balanced by a view that AIDS is a colonialist import.

Once the reservoir of infection can be identified, either by reference to high risk groups or, as was possible after 1985, by antibody testing, it is perhaps inevitable that there should be calls for the identification and segregation of the guilty (Altman, 1986: 63; Watney, 1988: 52). There have been restrictions on immigration and a great deal of talk of segregation, isolation and, most tellingly, of marking, branding individuals, making visible the invisible.

'Sentence First, Verdict Afterwards'

In 1989 Richard Goldstein wrote:

> Every time I heard about another death in the early stages of the epidemic, I would strain to find some basis for a distinction between the deceased and myself: he was a clone, a crisco queen, a midnight sling artist. . . . When it moved in on my friends, the epidemic shattered my presumption of immunity. I, too, was vulnerable, and everything I thought and did about AIDS changed once I faced that fact.' (Goldstein, 1989: 81)

The tendency, the need to locate the threat to oneself in 'the other' permeates AIDS discourse. But it would be wrong to suggest, even by omission, that this need is confined to those whose contribution to understanding the epidemic has been unhelpful: the political right, the tabloid press or the moral fascists. Even within the rapidly expanding volumes of articles dedicated to well-meaning attempts to understand and prevent the further spread of HIV, similar witch-hunts are all too common. As we shall have occasion to discuss at length in later chapters, the dominant paradigm of behavioural research on gay men has concentrated on identifying those who engage in unsafe sex.

This process shares many of the characteristics of the search for the homosexual or for the member of the risk group. Like them, the person who has unsafe sex (the PHUS) is deemed to be invisible, but identifiable by the arcane arts of forensic psychology or psychiatry. He is deemed to be a danger more to others than himself, to be dedicated to the seduction of the innocent or the unwary, whose resolve and skill in evading and resisting him must be bolstered by the provision of counselling and sessions on empowerment. He lurks always out there, somewhere in the dark and dangerous nether world of promiscuous sex, without commitment or care, to be challenged by the provision of knowledge, the fostering of appropriate attitudes and the inculcation of beliefs about the virus and its effects which accord with the grand rational project of the AIDS industry.

Over the decade in which AIDS has dominated our lives and decimated our communities, we seem dedicated to a bizarre dance in which the search for difference, the desire to discover the mark of the beast divides one from the other, renders us dubious of ourselves and distrustful of those we meet. The positivist project survives. As psychologists, sociologists, public health analysts, behavioural scientists of all sorts earnestly publish their earnest findings, seeing themselves perhaps as George Smiley, perhaps as Dr van Helsing, we seek the sallow cheek, the shadow beneath the eye, the glint of fear. By warning us always of the other, these scientists begin to erode the trust that articulates the gay community. We begin to distrust the young, the old, those who drink, those on drugs, those who come from America or travel to Amsterdam, those who are sluts or those we saw coming out of the clinic, those who go cruising or dancing or those into leather or bondage or 'cuffs, those who are forward, those who are shy, those who look foreign or those who are sleek and above all those who seem just a little odd. But most potently and perniciously, the search for the other distracts attention from the one place that he will always be found — the mirror.

Until, like Goldstein, we recognize and accept that we could become, might be, are already HIV positive, we will fail as individuals to have compassion with rather than sympathy for those whose suffering is greater than our own, fail as a community and as a nation to develop credible and workable care and prevention programs, fail as scientists to understand the true nature of the problem that we seek so earnestly to understand. By seeking elsewhere the unsafe individual, we delude ourselves.

The lesson is hardly novel or recent. Nigh on 3000 years ago King Oedipus sought the reason for the barrenness of his country. He was told that 'there is an unclean thing, born and nursed on our soil, polluting our soil, which must be driven away, not kept to destroy us.' He, like all his progeny and all his inheritors, sought the unclean thing throughout the land, only to be told finally: 'You are the cursed polluter of this land', 'the killer you are seeking is yourself.' He put out his own eyes in horrified recognition of his earlier wilful blindness. Let us not drive ourselves to that sorry end.

5 Theorising Sex

> Making love is like a dance. It requires intelligence to know what the other is going to do. He must understand the other person to bring out the best in him. (Anonymous interviewee quoted in Westwood, 1960: 118)

The past decade and the growth of the AIDS industry have seen advances in many fields of scientific research. In the behavioural sciences a challenge of the greatest importance has been the explanation of moves towards safer sex among gay and bisexual men and the maintenance of those changes over time. These changes have primarily been understood as health-promoting manoeuvres made by men at an individual level. Consequently, 'failure' to adopt safer sex has also been viewed at an individual level. Over the period of our research we have sought to develop an alternative approach to the understanding of sexual behaviour in general, and unsafe behaviour in particular. This model is theoretically informed, humanistic and holistic in scope and based on the simple insight that sex is interpersonal and interactive. In this chapter we sketch the tenets of the traditional approach, set out our criticisms of it, and in the final section set out our understanding of the interactional matrix within which sexual behaviour is negotiated and moulded.

The Traditional Account

While it is not always possible to do so when considering specific pieces of research, it is helpful to distinguish two broad families of theoretical model. The first is the Health Belief Model (HBM) which is a psychological formulation widely used in the study of health behaviour (Becker, 1974). The other is an approach deriving from the area of risk perception. These approaches are not logically incompatible and are often deployed in parallel (see, for example, Fitzpatrick *et al.*, 1989). While other models of risk behaviour have been, or are starting to be, considered, such as those grounded in social support (Prieur, 1990) or in unconscious neurotic motivations (Odets, 1992), the HBM and models based on risk perception have been by far the most common theoretical frameworks.

The Health Belief Model

The HBM is a model of decision-making that attempts to predict whether or not people will accept medical intervention and treatment, and whether they will follow prevention recommendations such as attending regular screenings, not smoking, or engaging in safer sex. It is based on two broad interacting bases. The first is the individual's willingness, readiness or preparedness to make the potentially health improving change. Factors affecting this willingness may include knowledge of the illness (its physical manifestations or how it is transmitted), an assessment of its seriousness (whether it is potentially fatal), and the cost involved in making the change (what you have to give up and how much you value that). The second, interactional factor is the structural or external factors that aid or hinder change, and include such things as the financial cost and the availability of peer support. Historically the HBM has been applied to a wide variety of health-related behaviour, and as such was an obvious model in trying to understand the move to safer sex. Thus a number of projects adopted the HBM as a model to work within, or attempted to develop the model as an explanatory framework.

Probably the best known HBM derivative model of safer sex is the AIDS Risk Reduction Model (Catania *et al.*, 1990). This model proposes three stages of change comprising '(1) recognition and labelling of one's sexual behaviours as high risk for contracting HIV, (2) making a commitment to reduce high risk sexual contacts and increase low risk activities and (3) seeking and enacting strategies to obtain these goals'(p. 54), The model thus posits a relationship between knowledge of, attitudes towards and beliefs about AIDS, HIV and safer sex and the uptake of safer sexual practices. Specifically, the model states that the desired outcome, safer sexual practices, will occur if and only if the practitioners *know* about and have positive *attitudes* towards safe sex and also *believe* that safe sex will have the desired effect.

What we might term the basic model is typically augmented in various ways, most importantly by the introduction of the concept of self-efficacy (Bandura, 1977) or internal locus of control (Rotter, 1966). Noting that knowledge, attitudes and beliefs are not sufficient to predict behaviour change, researchers sought the mediating factors which enhanced or impeded their ability to act on their wishes. The notion of self-efficacy derives from social learning theories (e.g., Seligman's (1975) theory of learned helplessness). It proposes that, dependent on the outcomes of individual action, especially those during childhood, people develop a sense of whether or not they are able to control what goes on around them. For example, a child who is praised and punished indiscriminately for what he or she does will learn that 'that's the way things go', and perceive themselves as being subject to the whims of fate. Alternatively, a child who is praised for doing good and punished for doing bad, will learn that outcomes are dependent on his or her actions, and consequently feel in control of the environment. Self-efficacy proposes that this perception consequently becomes self-fulfilling, and affects people's ability to 'take control of their own lives'. The notion has some surface validity in the area, say, of smoking.

The HBM potentiates what Aggleton (1989: 223) has described as the 'information giving' model of health education, the goal of which is 'to reduce the incidence of disease by bringing about changes in individual behaviour', a goal to be achieved by the provision of information. The popularity of the model can be at least partly explained by the fact that it focuses attention on processes which are relatively amenable to intervention: the provision of information, the fostering of positive attitudes towards safe sex and of negative attitudes towards unsafe behaviour, and the promulgation of the simple message that safe sex works. The model also has a commonsense intuitive appeal.

Models of Risk Assessment

The second major strand of theoretical modelling of the uptake and maintenance of safer sex derives from ideas about subjective risk assessment (Kahneman and Tversky, 1972; Tversky and Kahneman, 1974). The assessment of risk is a complex facet of human life driven by fear or anxiety of uncertain outcomes. Fear and anxiety are complex and sensitive biological mechanisms that generate motivation for the coping actions that are a natural consequence of risk assessments. Hence, faced with a situation involving events whose consequences are undesirable and whose future occurrence is uncertain, individuals make an assessment of two things: the probability of an adverse outcome given a certain course of action; and the seriousness of the potential outcome.

Thus, faced by the threat of HIV, people have to judge the probability of infection, either from a given sexual encounter or from their sexual lifestyle in general, and the effect this would have on their well-being. While most individuals may be adept at making such judgments, these processes are notoriously difficult to quantify, not least because they often, in practice, affect one another in the sense that a particularly serious outcome will be seen as more likely than a less serious one.

Within this approach there are two broad schools. On the one hand, the straightforward risk assessment model sees the problem as one of convincing men that there is a real probability of infection. This focuses attention on 'perceived invulnerability' or, famously, 'denial'. Implicit in this approach is the idea that the consequences of HIV infection are so bad that no-one would rationally discount them, though this has taken something of a knock with the discovery of 'survivor guilt' (Odets, 1992). The second broad strand of risk assessment models is the 'cost-benefit' analysis of sexual behaviour. In this model the costs of adopting safer sex in terms of the loss of pleasure have to be counted against the benefits of non-infection. While there is much to be said for this approach, the way in which it has traditionally been used (see, for example, McKusick *et al.*, 1985) is to call for the eroticisation of safer sex — of condoms, of body rubbing — in an attempt to minimise the difference in pleasure to be gained from safe as opposed to unsafe behaviour. In risk assessment models the decision process is often represented as a choice, either to fuck or not to do so. Each choice carries with it a probability of becoming infected with HIV (if currently uninfected) or of passing it on (if currently infected). There are thus four possible outcomes: (1) fucking and passing the virus; (2) fucking and not passing the virus; (3) not fucking and passing the virus; and (4) not fucking and not passing the virus. Each of the four outcomes has a unique utility to the individual which is a function of three values: the utility of infection; the utility of the fuck; and the probability of infection. The rational man or woman will choose the outcome with the greatest utility.

Approaches that concentrate on individuals' risk assessments lie behind Aggleton's (1989: 223) second model of health education, 'self-empowerment', in which the goal is the enhancement of 'people's ability to act rationally rather than on the basis of emotions and feelings', a goal to be achieved by 'participatory learning, group work and self-exploration to help clients identify the choices they can make.'

Some Problems with the Traditional Accounts

The models outlined above contain two fallacious assumptions. First, they overlook a simple and obvious fact: that all sex in which HIV may be transmitted involves more than one person, and, consequently, that the behaviour can neither be understood nor accounted for by looking at one person alone. We have termed this assumption the individualist fallacy (Davies *et al.*, 1992). The second assumption entrenched in these models concerns the way we think about sex and how it fits into our lives (or how researchers think about their sex and how it fits into their lives). In particular it regards the practice of safer sex as a process of control, specifically a process of rational control of the animal urges. Since this builds on ideas associated with the romantic movement, we have termed it the romantic fallacy (Davies *et al.*, 1992).

The Individualist Fallacy

The vast majority of articles on unsafe sex among gay and bisexual men seek to elucidate the reasons why individuals continue to have unsafe sex. They aim to enable the identification of individuals and groups who are in need of intervention, in the form of education, therapy or support. This search has two dubious features: its concentration on individual traits, and its assumption that these traits must be deficiencies of one sort or another. The concentration on the individual betrays a naive psychology. We are being asked to believe that individuals carry around with them fixed propensities for unsafe behaviour, and the assumption that unsafe sex is to be explained by deficiencies of one sort or another is a form of the positivist heritage that we have commented on in Chapter 1.

This focus on the individual is fundamentally misguided. Sex is, after language, the most interpersonal of human activities. It is, in its myriad diversities, an exchange of pleasure, a negotiation of desire, a sharing of self and body. The progress of a sexual session is a physical conversation, within which intercourse may play an important role (or it may not), with different meaning and connotation in different circumstances. Men engage in anal intercourse (or not) as a result of an ongoing, explicit or implicit negotiation between (at least) two individuals.

It is true that the paradigm models of risk reduction usually incorporate some measure of communication skill, but two problems render this inclusion spurious and ultimately unhelpful. First, the measures explicitly or implicitly (implicit often in the illustrative material which accompanies the analysis) assume that the negotiation of safer sex is verbal. It seems to be assumed that the conversation: 'Shall we use a condom, then?' 'Yeh, why not', is the limit of 'negotiation'. The majority of communication in sex is non-verbal. That this is possible is obvious if we concede that two men, who share no common language, can have sex together, or that men can have sex without exchanging words. If language were crucial to the negotiation process, we might expect these sexual sessions never to get off the ground. This is obviously not the case. Each sexual session is the result of a negotiation which continues from before the physical connection is made to the post-coital cigarette.

Second, while an individual can be thought to have better or worse communication skills, it is surely inappropriate to suppose that they will always be able equally to put them into practice. Within a given relationship an individual will find themself sometimes in control of the situation, at other times under the control of their partner. It is important to recognise that sexual negotiation, while universal, is not necessarily between *equals*. Age differences, racial differences, disparities in social or economic status, sexual attractiveness, sexual role, etc. all create sexual situations in which one individual becomes more able to dictate the course of events than the other, though these abilities are not fixed, even between two individuals. Communication skills are not static (as the usually calm converser who freezes in front of an audience will confirm). They change over time, with different people and with the same people in different situations.

This is not to say that individuals do not hold knowledge, attitudes and beliefs towards HIV on a personal level, and that these will not affect their sexual behaviour. They clearly will. What we suggest is mistaken is the assumption that you can use this information to predict their sexual behaviour in each and every circumstance, irrespective of the characteristics, beliefs, attitudes and knowledge of their partner and the circumstances the pair find themselves in. Concentrating on aspects of an individual can tell us no more than half the story of a particular sexual encounter, and it is most unlikely to tell us this much, because it tells us nothing about either the partner's individual characteristics or the interaction between partners.

The Romantic Fallacy

Not only do the dominant models of unsafe sex concentrate on the individual to an unwarranted and unhelpful extent; they also perpetuate the notion that sex is 'natural', overwhelming and supremely irrational (or at best non-rational). Two millennia of Christian thought have deeply ingrained in the Western mind a belief in the subservience of the body to the will and have led to the belief that the body's demands — lust, thirst, pleasure, etc. — are undesirable, evil and subhuman drives. This idea is reinforced by the romantic tradition, with its characterisation of love as an overwhelming passion over which one has no control (hence falling in love; love will find a way; love conquers all) and which cannot be denied.

In the dominant paradigm, unsafe sexual behaviour, especially fucking without a condom, is seen as a basic (irrational) drive which the (rational) will is constantly striving to control. Prieur's (1990) important work on the meaning of fucking to gay men emphasises the naturalness of the experience. Safer sex is seen as a necessary but unpleasant course of action which is dictated by prudence rather than desire (Pollak, 1988). We may distinguish two corollaries of this attitude which are of particular moment. First, it is assumed that safer sex is *the* rational choice. No-one could possibly *choose* to have unsafe sex or make a conscious and reasoned decision to fuck. This fallacy rests on a fundamental misunderstanding of the term 'rational', which we shall take up below. Second, it leads to a conception of safer sex as a strategy of control, both at the individual level and, by extension, at the social, normative level. In particular, monogamy features as a preferred response to HIV/AIDS, and a distressing number of recent papers and contributions bury this moral agenda in their criteria of 'unsafe sex'. Third, the goal of the paradigm model seems to be the eradication of fucking among gay men. Quite apart from the homophobia which this attitude displays, it is an impractical and undesirable goal, for reasons which we now examine.

Some Considerations for a Model of Sexual Behaviour

The notion of rationality lies at the heart of the debate about safer sexual practice. Yet the concept is often used in a contradictory and confusing manner, which muddies the debate and is unhelpful in the urgent task of understanding, establishing and reinforcing safer sexual behaviour. Perhaps the most insidious and pervasive misuse of the term 'rational' is that which confuses the process of decision-making with the decision itself. When used correctly, the term refers to the process, not the outcome. Thus a decision is rational if it is made after a consideration of the available evidence in the light of the circumstances pertaining at the time. By contrast, an irrational decision is one which ignores, dismisses or otherwise deems irrelevant available information. The eventual decision — which we will take, for the sake of exemplar and without loss of generality, to be a decision to fuck — may, in addition, be right or wrong according to epidemiological or other criteria, but the rationality of the decision process is independent of the rightness of the outcome. Thus an individual can (1) rationally come to the right decision; (2) irrationally come to the right decision; (3) rationally come to the wrong decision; (4) irrationally come to the wrong decision. The criteria on which we decide whether a decision is right or wrong and the criteria by which we decide if a process is rational or irrational are distinct.

Rationality and Heuristic

Even among those writers who use 'rational' to refer to the process of decision-making, there is a tendency to use an unrealistically complex version of the decision-making process. They regard individuals as making rational decisions on the basis of detailed epidemiological data and sophisticated models of contagion and infection which are simply outside the scope of the ordinary person in the street or bedroom.

A common assumption of researchers using the rational model is that the utility of infection, or more accurately its disutility, is so overwhelming that the transient pleasure of a mere fuck cannot, rationally, ever outweigh the potential devastation of infection. This is a bloodless and arrogant view, yet it underpins the agenda which sees the eradication of HIV transmission as following from the eradication of fucking among gay men. Where the choice is starkest, say among street children, it is surely an entirely rational decision to be fucked if the alternative is to starve. Having said that, the choice between the possibility of a slow death in a number of years and the certainty of death now is one which all of us should be ashamed to impose on anyone. To add to that the arrogance of dismissing the validity of choice is inexcusable.

Third, the failure of the model as a descriptive tool lies in its elision of the fact that individuals make choices not on the basis of accurate information — your average man in the cottage does not anxiously peruse the *British Medical Journal* to assess the prevalence of HIV infection in his locality, but on the basis of heuristic rules (Tversky and Kahneman, 1974; Weatherburn, 1990). Thus the common decision in the early years of the epidemic in Britain not to fuck with Americans was a relatively good heuristic device which recognised the difference in prevalence between the two countries. On the other hand, cues such as the physical appearance of an individual or his perceived lifestyle are relatively poor heuristic devices and are rightly discouraged by health promotion interventions.

Externally, as it were, the agreement to have sex forms part of the ongoing dialogue between two (or more) individuals. This dialogue might be brief and predicated upon the expectation of sex (the casual partner) or part of a long, subtle and multi-stranded discussion (the long-term relationship). Within either of these dialogues the sexual encounter may have any number of specific meanings, often more than one in any one encounter: I fancy you; I love you: I hate you; I forgive you; do you love me; you are special, etc. Internally the structure of the encounter will have its own logic or grammar which will carry certain other messages which may confirm or confuse the main message of the encounter. It is the protean nature of this relationship which has ensured its avoidance by the analyst. The imperatives of AIDS urge its understanding.

In conclusion, then, let us summarise. The tendency in discussions of unsafe sexual behaviour has been attempts to isolate the characteristics of those individuals who engage in these activities. However, more recently, attempts have been made to elicit and explain the symbolic meanings of sexual acts — particularly unsafe acts — leaving open the path for a theory of sexual behaviour in an epidemic which emphasises the rational aspects of individuals' choices. Our contention is that this theory requires a sustained and serious examination of dyadic sexual communication in order to succeed in moulding together what are now very disparate bits of information. It is to the beginning of such an examination that we now turn.

The SIGMA Model

As we have indicated above, the SIGMA model derives from the simple insight that unsafe sex involves at least two individuals. This leads us to focus attention not on the unsafe individual and his problems, but on the unsafe encounter or session, and to seek to understand the dynamics of sexual action within encounters in general and unsafe encounters in particular.

We put forward a number of theses concerning sexual behaviour which are basic to our understanding of sexual behaviour in general and unsafe sex in particular.

- Sexual behaviour is learned.

We assert that, far from being a natural, instinctual process, having sex is a learnt behaviour. We all, whatever our sexual preference or proclivity, go through a learning process about sexual behaviour which may include formal school sex education, informal information gained from family, peers and the media, watching others engage (either in films or in actuality) and practical experience (Thomson and Scott, 1991). Indeed, if we are lucky, our sexual careers are long-term learning processes, learning to experience pleasure in different ways from different parts of the body and from different stimuli.

- The learning of sex is like the learning of a language.

We do not learn to have sex in the same way as we learn to tie our shoelaces. It is not a simple action which, once learned, we simply repeat when and where appropriate. Rather, we learn sex like we learn a language. We learn a set of techniques which we then use creatively and dynamically and in many different ways. As in the use of language, the meaning that can attach to 'the same' act or sequence of acts will differ from person to person and from situation to situation. However, the basic vocabulary of sex is, compared to that of the English language, relatively limited. Whereas the number of words in English is in the hundreds of thousands, the number of sexual acts or techniques is probably to be numbered in the dozens. But, as in language, the potential for neologisms is immense. As we invent words to reflect the growing complexity of our world, so we can sexualise actions to increase and diversify the range and complexity of our pleasure.

- Having sex is like having a conversation.

To extend the analogy, it is helpful, we believe, to consider a sexual encounter as a conversation: a negotiation of meaning between two or more individuals. In the same way as a conversation can have different tones, different dynamics, different outcomes, so can a sexual conversation evoke different feelings and different reactions and meanings — even if it consists of the 'same' basic acts. Again, as some conversations become arguments and others are interrupted by the telephone or become repetitive, so sexual sessions can carry overtones of violence, be interrupted or degenerate into a boring and predictable sequence of acts and moves. Some conversations and sexual sessions can be long, deep and fulfilling, others can be unsatisfactory and yet others can be complete disasters in which misunderstandings are generated.

- Knowing how is different from knowing why.

We engage in a large number of conversations every day and we are all more or less competent at doing so. Certainly, some individuals find all conversations difficult or anxiety-provoking. All of us have been involved in conversations that we would rather leave. But most of us are able to participate in conversations, because we know how to do so. (The last sentence is, of course, a tautology.) We are not, however, able in the same way to explain the 'rules' of conversation. By this we do not mean the dictates of taste and manners that might engage the pen of a Barbara Cartland, but the complex rules which govern who speaks when, about what and why. For example, one simple rule of conversation is 'one at a time'. Conversation analysts have shown that the a pause of some fraction of a second gives an indication that an utterance has ended. We *know that* it is our turn to speak, but we do not *know why* we know that it is. In the same way we know how to have sex, but find it far more difficult to say why we did so. It is because of this difficulty of saying why something has happened in a sexual session that lies behind the idea that sex is natural and irrational.

- Fucking is an important but not universal part of the language of sex.

In Chapter 11 we will show some of the salience which fucking has for different men. It is important and sufficient to note here that fucking will carry different meanings, connotations and implications for the same men in different circumstances: with different partners, in different contexts, in different places.

- Unsafe sex can be thought of as an argument.

We have all known conversations that degenerate into arguments. In some cases this is due to the bloody-mindedness of one of the participants. In other cases it is the flow of the conversation that has led, seemingly inexorably, to the argument. In yet other cases it appears to have arisen almost spontaneously. Sometimes, indeed, individuals begin a conversation in order to have an argument. The important point here is that it takes two to argue. Both participants have, in a sense, to agree to argue.

Likewise, both participants in a sexual session must agree in some sense to have unsafe sex (we exclude rape in this instance). It may be that one of them was more responsible than the other, or that one was more weak-willed or persuasive or bloody-minded. But the decision was a joint one and both are responsible. By making the analogy with argument, we should emphasise that we are not seeing unsafe sex always as a failure. Unsafe sex eventuates from the decisions taken by a pair of individuals in a particular circumstance. As it is sometimes said that 'there was no alternative' to argument or that a quarrel was a healthy occurrence, so unsafe sex can emerge from good and honourable motives. Although usually dismissed by hard-line scientists, statements such as, 'I wanted to please him' or 'It seemed like the right thing to do' are not wimpish excuses but potent reasons. In the same way, therefore, that a theory of argument would have to take into account the possibility that individuals sometimes want to avoid argument, yet find themselves embroiled, so a theory of unsafe sex has to take into account the ways in which the learnt logic of the sexual session can overcome agreements reached prior to the session.

- Unsafe sex is not irrational, but a different sort of rationality.

Some men may have unsafe sex in a session despite their earlier conviction not to do so. We suggest that this is not necessarily due to a failure of rationality, but to the logic of the sexual conversation dominating over the logic of safety. Thus, our assessment of the costs and benefits of engaging in safer sex will vary according to the context we find ourselves in: in the midst of a particularly steamy session we may decide the immediate rewards of a decision are far more important than the long-term (potential) costs. This is not necessarily irrational.

Let us be quite clear about the analogy that we are drawing between unsafe sex and argument. First, we are *not* saying that it is possible to decide in a particular situation that one person is right and the other wrong. We are not concerned with the content of the argument, but with the process. Thus unsafe sex is like an argument in that:

1 it requires two individuals to engage. It is simply not possible for one person to have an argument by himself. It takes two to argue, as it takes two to have unsafe sex.
2 one person may indeed be more to 'blame' for the starting of the argument, but the other must respond, and this is as great a responsibility. Not answering, not agreeing to have sex is as much a decision as answering back, going along with the suggestion of unsafe behaviour. In a conversation I always have the option of walking away, of refusing to argue, of pushing the conversation in other ways. In the same way, I always have the option of refusing the proffered uncovered penis, of leaving the sexual encounter, of doing something that takes his mind off the unsafe sex. This is my absolute responsibility and, if I choose to argue, if I choose to engage in unsafe sex, then that is my responsibility, not my partner's. The option of withdrawal from argument is always open. We can walk away, refuse to proceed, but most of us feel obliged to continue, for reasons of pride, pig-headedness or simply because we have become immersed in the process. Similarly, the option to stop unsafe sex exists at each and every second of an encounter, even after it has begun. Many will feel obliged to continue, for reasons of pride, refusal to offend or simply because they are caught up in the moment.
3 in some cases an argument comes about despite the best intentions of the individuals involved. Like conversations, sexual sessions have an internal logic, and just as some conversations appear to lead inexorably towards argument, some sexual sessions will appear to move towards unsafe sex. Both individuals in a sexual encounter may have no prior intention to have unsafe sex, but the point in the proceedings may come when it seems the right, the logical, the natural thing to do. We suggest that it is in these cases that the branding of individuals as incapable, as deficient, as lacking in will or good sense is not only inappropriate but actually harmful in deflecting attention away from the important issues.
4 in other cases it comes about because both want it to. Sometimes a good argument is productive. It allows individuals to say things which might have been festering; it allows a free and frank interchange of opinions that might otherwise have been hidden. In the same way, there are good reasons for having unsafe sex. (We take up this point in the next section of this chapter.)
5 there may, indeed, be individuals who are argumentative, in the same way as there may be individuals who are suckers for argument. This account recognises the possibility that there are individuals who might be looking for unsafe sex more than others: those who find it so exciting or fulfilling or necessary that they seek it in every or many encounters. In the same way, there may be those whose personalities make them relative pushovers when it comes to demands for unsafe sex.

6 in the same way that it would be foolish of any one of us to say that he will never have an argument again, so is it foolish to deny the possibility of ever having unsafe sex.

The Terms of the Model

We suggest that each sexual session is a complex creative process in which power and pleasure, safety and danger, love and lust are negotiated and expressed. To make this clearer, we distinguish four logically distinct facets:

1 the two individuals;
2 the interaction between them;
3 the scenario or psychic context; and
4 the physical context.

We discuss these in detail below, but it is worth noting here that we are trying to describe in static terms a session which is a dynamic event, a process of some complexity in the course of which the meaning it has for each of the participants, the emotions, feelings and intentions they each experience will change from moment to moment.

The Individuals

Individuals bring with them to the sexual conversation a range of beliefs, feelings and ideas about sex which are relatively fixed and others which are more fluid and amenable to alteration in particular circumstances. As we shall see in Chapter 11, there are some men for whom anal intercourse is a central, perhaps indispensable part of sex. Others feel that the imperative of safe sex precludes anal intercourse in almost any circumstances. Most men, we suggest, balance these views. Even so, it will not be the case that every time the man with the clear safer sex beliefs has sex, he will have safe sex, nor will the man who is excited above all else by anal intercourse always engage. These needs and/or desires will be mediated by the interaction with his partner before and during the sexual session.

Other aspects of the individual are relevant, such as his gender identity, his expectations of what constitutes 'sex', past experience of particular sexual techniques and how long it is since he last had sex. These relatively fixed items of the individual's personality are accompanied by others which vary more quickly. Some individuals are prone to depression, during which their commitment to safer sex may flag. Others may be anxious and become almost phobic about fucking. All of us have moods which may alter our feelings about unsafe sex, irrespective of the context or interaction. This is an important contention, for it seeks to locate within us all the potential for unsafe sex, rather than in *them*, a group to be described by *our* science (cf. Chapter 4).

Some versions of the traditional account accept that depression, anxiety or other mood states might affect the propensity of individuals to have unsafe sex. Yet they typically treat these as fixed parts of the individual's make-up. For example, consider a man who has hitherto had safe sex who finds himself in a situation where he has lost his job, or his flat, or his boyfriend or any combination of these, and therefore, or for any other reason, has become depressed and cares not about his future. If he then has unsafe sex, we may from our viewpoint regard this as unfortunate or dangerous. Indeed, some time later, he may regret or even be frightened by what he has done. But his need is not as the traditional account suggests for further education about safer sex. It is for help in clearing the depression, or help in finding a job or flat.

The Interaction

As each sexual session begins, each partner will have a set of expectations or hopes about what will happen. These may be quite vague or quite explicit. They may have been verbally negotiated beforehand. They may be the result of experience, as in a long-term relationship, where each knows the likely course of events, sometimes with great boredom. Even in the case of the casual encounter, expectations are set up by physical appearance, clothing, body posture, facial expression, or by a sophisticated system of signs such as coloured handkerchiefs.

We have noted above that one of the subjects of the sexual conversation is power, but the issue in the understanding of unsafe sex is the issue of control. The man in control of the session is not necessarily the one who is in the 'masculine' role. Control is mediated by social factors: greater age, greater financial power, greater experience will all tend to invest some individuals with control. But these will be pitted against each other in the sexual negotiation, and these can change from session to session even between the same individuals. Consider the following. A middle-aged, relatively wealthy man of mediocre attractiveness may meet a young, good-looking but relatively impoverished man and have sex. In this relationship the older man may seek to assert control through his greater age, experience and material wealth. He may be hampered in this, however, by his realisation of the young man's greater currency in the sexual marketplace. The older man may then cede control of the session to the younger to ensure that the session is a success from his (the younger man's) perspective in the hope that the relationship will continue. If it does so, however, the balance will subtly shift. Once the younger man has indicated his continuing attraction or perhaps his commitment to a longer relationship, the balance of control shifts. As a relationship develops, the balance of play between the two will become more complex. As arguments develop and fade, as the two get to know each other better, as a host of contingent matters impinges upon them, so will the capital that each brings to a session vary. Sex does not just happen. It occurs because two men want it to, for any one of a host of reasons.

Scenario

Together, the participants in a sexual session seek to create an erotically charged atmosphere. This may be done through physical paraphernalia or through psychic means. These psychic scenes or scenarios may be more or less overt, more or less rigid. A scenario need not be shared. One participant may be lying there pretending to be the Queen of Sheba and getting off on it, while his partner is unaware.

To the extent that the scenario is verbally negotiated, it may be more or less sophisticated. It may, at one extreme, involve a game of, say, trucker and hitch-hiker in which the playing out of a phantasmagorical sequence of events constrains the interaction tightly. At the other extreme, a single whispered compliment or command such as 'Ride me, cowboy' will set up a momentary frame of psychic reference which may enhance the erotic charge of the encounter. On the other hand, a mischosen word can lead to the session dissolving in giggles.

In some cases these scenarios may have been worked out in detail before the session began. Conversations, sometimes over the telephone, describing the proposed session themselves give vicarious excitement. Others emerge unbidden from the interaction itself. It is possible that the scenario will involve anal intercourse as an integral part of its action. For example, the couple who are seeking to mimic or reproduce the action of a sexually explicit video will have to make a decision whether to fuck as they do on the film. Other scenarios may be built which exclude anal intercourse.

There is potential for a scenario to build towards unsafe sex, if we take that to mean sex that the individuals involved would not otherwise choose to engage in. The logic of the action might drive to a conclusion in which one of the participants is fucked unmercifully. In this situation the participants are faced with a choice: to explore the scenario to its end, or to innovate to exclude the unsafe behaviour. Their ability to do this will depend on their skill and imagination. It is not, however, an irrational process. It is one in which choices are made and over which there is rational control. To the extent that the action of the scenario is pre-specified, then the potential for it to develop in unexpected ways is limited (though not, of course, eradicated). Pre-specification therefore guards against unsafe sex, but only to an extent.

Context

A sexual session can gain in meaning and significance from its physical context. In some cases this may be negligible, as when a couple have sex in the same bedroom that they have used for the past twenty years. One is unlikely to be turned on by this context, even if the wall-paper is changed. On the other hand, a quick grope in the back of a bus or in a public place can, because of the context, create a significant erotic charge.

The gay scene includes some very specific sexual contexts, as we shall see in Chapter 10. Some of these are more conducive to certain forms of sex than others. Cottages or other places where members of the public might impinge are not, in general, conducive to fucking but rather encourage forms of sex which allow quick disengagement. Others allow norms of safer sex to be maintained, sometimes explicitly as in 'jack-off clubs' or safe sex parties.

Safer Sex as Strategy

We have so far concentrated on the understanding of safer sex as a tactical issue, that is at the level of the individual encounter. In this section we examine the ways in which safer sex has become part of the strategic concern of men in the decade or more since AIDS appeared.

Early health promotion exercises, including those of the Terrence Higgins Trust (see Chapter 3) concentrated on the identification and elimination of particular unsafe practices. As it became clearer that anal intercourse was by far the most risky of activities, so campaigns focused on reducing or even eradicating anal intercourse among gay and bisexual men. Similar moves to discourage sucking faded as the evidence grew that the practice was relatively safe. Thus it can be seen that what counts as safer sex has changed over the last decade, even in the views of 'experts'.

Among 'ordinary' gay men too, understandings have changed. Since the beginning of our work in 1987, we have seen an increase in the general level of sexual activity. More men are having more sex with more people. We have interpreted this increase as the result of a growing confidence among our cohort about the imperatives of safer sex. We think that in the earlier years of the project many men continued to avoid sex in all its forms as a means of ensuring their safety. As time has passed, the number of men who do this has declined and more are now having sex again. As part of this change, the number of partners with whom fucking occurred has also increased, though not as fast as the number of partners. In this sense, anal intercourse is becoming more common. The question remains, however: is this increase to be understood as an increase in unsafe sex?

Kippax *et al.* (1992) have defined unsafe sex as 'practices which, independent of the context in which they occur, carry a high probability of HIV transmission.' They recognise that all acts of unprotected anal intercourse are not equally unsafe. This point is accepted by most, if not all, researchers. The question that divides them is where the boundary between safe and unsafe should be drawn. The problem is that there is a conflict between the need of researchers to construct a straightforward criterion of unsafe sex and the experience of individuals making decisions about their own behaviour from day to day. What seems to have happened is that researchers have constructed such unitary measures primarily for their own convenience and then explicitly or implicitly used those same criteria to judge the behaviour of groups and to prescribe the behaviour of individuals. For example, the San Francisco group CAPS uses a criterion of unsafe sex which is 'unprotected anal intercourse with a non-monogamous partner' (Ekstrand, Stall *et al.*, 1992). As epidemiological criteria go, this is a fairly accurate aggregate measure. It is certainly to be preferred to others such as 'visiting a GUM clinic' or 'meeting a prostitute', both of which have featured as measures of unsafe sex but neither of which carries a great deal of intrinsic risk.

The problem arises when this simple criterion is used to prescribe behaviour; when it becomes the focus of health education campaigns; when such campaigns are demanded on the basis of 'high' levels of unsafe sex and when they are then focused on eliminating such behaviour. We believe that such simplistic approaches to understanding sexual behaviour not only insult the sophistication of the men they seek to address, but are also counter-productive in proscribing behaviour which may be safe and reinforcing behaviour which may not be.

The key to understanding this problem is the acceptance that no single act of anal intercourse is absolutely safe. Each carries with it a varying amount of risk. In some cases this risk is so small that most would agree that it can be discounted. This might be the case if a couple had been monogamous since before the start of the epidemic, or neither had had penetrative sex before. In other cases it would be generally agreed that some encounters are extremely risky. Repeated sessions including unprotected anal intercourse between a couple with known and discordant serostatus is undeniably risky. Between these extremes, however, is a range of situations where the state of affairs is less clear-cut and where most men make most of their decisions most of the time.

We assert that many men make strategic decisions about the risks they are prepared to take in their sexual lives and that (1) they come to different decisions on the level of acceptable risk, and (2) they do so with imperfect knowledge. The aim of behavioural science in the study of such decisions is to recognise these processes and to incorporate them into their models and prescriptions for intervention.

Levels of Risk

As the preceding chapter has, we hope, made clear, we believe that making decisions about risk is a process that never forecloses. Men do not carry with them a pre-specified level of risk which is with them in the same way that their eye colour or the size of their genitalia is fixed, nor even in the way that their political preference is relatively fixed. Rather, that assessment is made about a particular session with a particular partner in a particular context.

Over time, men may come to different decisions about their behaviour. Some may routinely engage in behaviour which others will find unacceptably risky. The traditional account would label the former group as defective in some sense. We believe that this is an unacceptable ethical judgment. It is an ethical, not a scientific judgment because it involves an assessment not of what is the case — that different people make different judgments — but an assessment of what ought to be the case — what course of action is right or wrong. It is unacceptable because there is no absolute criterion of right and wrong in this case. By indicating a particular set of actions to be right and another set to be unsafe and wrong, the decisions are being divorced from their context and thereby stripped of the very information that is needed in order to judge their appropriateness.

Imperfect Information

Decisions in the real world are usually made without full knowledge either of the circumstances or of the consequences. All decisions about safe and unsafe sex involve, in the last analysis, a modicum of trust. Even in the case cited above, that of a couple living monogamously for over a decade, each partner has to trust that the other is indeed 'faithful', a judgment that is always based on belief rather than knowledge. In other cases different amounts of belief and trust are involved. Assessing the level of that belief is not possible in the abstract. Different people in the same circumstances and the same people in differing circumstances make differing judgments about the amount of information they need and the concomitant degree of trust they are willing to extend. It is not possible to decide what an acceptable degree of certainty is or might be — nor would it be helpful even if it could be.

Many of the criteria of unsafe sex preferred by researchers carry implicit moral overtones. The preference for monogamous relationships is at base a moral

Table 5.1. Risk Reduction Strategies

Strategy	Regular partner	Casual partners
1	No anal intercourse	No anal intercourse
2	No anal intercourse	Anal intercourse with condom
3	No anal intercourse	Anal intercourse no condom
4	Anal intercourse no condom	No anal intercourse
5	Anal intercourse no condom	Anal intercourse with condom
6	Anal intercourse no condom	Anal intercourse no condom
7	Anal intercourse with condom	No anal intercourse
8	Anal intercourse with condom	Anal intercourse with condom
9	Anal intercourse with condom	Anal intercourse no condom

one. Monogamous relationships do not guarantee safety. Rather, the degree of safety will depend, among other things, on the length of the relationship, the serostatus of the partners, the types of sexual activities involved and so on. As we have mentioned above, all this will also be mediated by the degree of trust that exists between the partners, a degree which will change over time.

In the more common situation (see Chapter 10) of open relationships, Table 5.1 shows the logical possibilities of risk reduction strategies adopted by gay and bisexual men. The criterion of unsafe sex as 'unprotected anal intercourse with a non-monogamous partner' includes a range of these behaviours, some of which have a greater degree of 'negotiated safety' than others. The point is that these represent different degrees of risk reduction, from strategy 1, which is probably the safest, to strategy 6, which is probably the least safe. Within these bounds, however, we suggest that men will make strategic decisions about the type(s) of sex that they will have in order to minimise the risks they run, if it is not possible to eliminate risk entirely. In this, they are acting in the same way as we all do all of the time. Driving a car, crossing the road, eating eggs, smoking cigarettes all carry risks which many people decide to take. The choice in these situations is a choice among strategies of risk reduction, not an attempt to live risk-free.

6 Approaches and Methods

Goe and catche a falling star,
    Get with child a mandrake roote,
Tell me where all the past yeares are,
    Or who cleft the Divels foote,
Teach me to heare Mermaldes singing,
    Or to keep off envies stinging
        And finde
        What winde
Serves to advance an honest minde

(John Donne)

The methods mentioned by John Donne in his anguished quest for true knowledge were, no doubt, quaint and exotic, even in his own day. Today, 300 years or so later, they reek of an unenlightened antiquity. In 300 years from now, perhaps the methods that we have at our disposal will seem equally fanciful, yet we must make do with those that are available.

The investigation and analysis of sexual behaviour involve many difficulties. The most central involves the imposition of categories on sexual actions. These categories arise from those used in everyday life, but in order that they be useful for a descriptive text such as this, it is necessary to be clearer about the exact reference than is the case in everyday conversation (see also Wellings *et al.*, 1990). We, therefore, begin with a description of the main units of analysis.

Units of Analysis

Although the perspective of the project places sexual behaviour within the context of general lifestyle, sexual behaviour was and remains the primary focus of our investigations. While there are those who will persist in seeing this as a reductionist approach, reminiscent of the medical models from before 1970, this is quite mistaken. At the heart of Project SIGMA's approach is a detailed analysis of the structure of sexual behaviour, which is notable for focusing attention not on the individual but on the process of sexual interaction, an approach which is invaluable in avoiding some of the pitfalls of the individualist fallacy (see Chapter 5). We believe that an analysis of the reaction of gay and bisexual men to HIV must build on an understanding of sexual behaviour in general.

Sexual Acts

The logical primitives of any study of sexual behaviour are, we suggest, sexual acts, not identities, proclivities or preferences. From the specific point of view of HIV, this focus is crucial since each act carries a different probability of transmitting the virus. From the general point of view, the formulation allows the complexity of sexual behaviour to be captured far more easily than approaches which begin with the individual.

The project identifies a set of fourteen core sexual acts: masturbation, fellatio, anal intercourse, anilingus, anodigital insertion, anobrachial intercourse, lindinism (urolagnia), coprophilia, enemas, frottage, inter-femoral intercourse, corporal punishment, massage and deep kissing. A number of points need to be made. First, although the list is long, it is not exhaustive. Other specific acts will be reported by individuals, whose range and the consequent length of the list of acts is limited only by inventiveness and physical ingenuity. Second, and more specifically, there are some acts which will always, in our culture at least, be considered sexual. The insertion of the penis into the rectum, for example, will always carry sexual connotations. On the other hand, there are acts which become sexual only because they occur in an erotic, sexualized context. Massage, for example, can carry little or no erotic charge on some occasions, while on others it might be intensely erotic. Third, by asserting the logical primacy of sexual acts, we are not engaged in a biological or behavioural reductionism. We are not seeking to confine these acts within sterile behavioural definitions. We are not, for example, saying that male masturbation is reducible to the stroking of an erect penis by the hand. Such an act becomes masturbation only when the actor so wills and understands it. The intention to masturbate gives the act meaning. These three points — infinity, contextuality and intentionality — point to the fact that the exercise in which we are engaged in this chapter is a refinement of thought, not a confinement of experience. Fourth, although it is in the nature of language to impose a logical framework on a fluid reality, it is not always possible to distinguish completely and absolutely the boundaries between acts. When does a massage of the genital area move to become a gentle masturbation? Does running the mouth and tongue along the shaft of the penis count as sucking? Just how much hand has to be inserted to count as fisting? We believe that these questions are not only unanswerable in the abstract, but also miss the point; the point being that actions become sexual in context, in the mind.

Gendering of Acts

It is clear that sexual acts are asymmetric in the sense that doing *x* to someone is not the same as having *x* done to you. One way to capture this asymmetry is to consider acts from the point of view of an ego, the actor. It is then possible to modulate each of the acts above, so that it can be done (1) by and to the self, (2) by the self to another, (3) by another to the self, and (4) by the self to another and by another to the self simultaneously. This device forms the basis of the project's sexual behaviour inventory and is used specifically in the diary method.[1] In principle, therefore, using the fourteen acts above, 4×14 modulated acts are defined, but some of these are physically impossible so the actual number is somewhat reduced (though not by as many as was originally thought; ingenuity and dexterity are quite amazing).

Some of these modulated acts can be gendered, either physically or psychically. Some modulated acts are possible only between a man and a woman, such as penile penetration of the vagina. Other acts which are not so confined are also gendered if, for example, they can be done 'by' a man 'to' a woman and by a man to a man, but not by a woman to a man.[2] In the latter case, we propose that the gender significance of the act remains when the act is performed in a homosexual context. Thus a woman may suck a man's penis, but a man may not do this to a woman. We suggest that the gendering of the act is also present when a man sucks another man's penis, though this does not necessarily mean that the suckee automatically becomes the feminine, only that this is a symbolic connotation that may be enhanced, subverted or transcended.

Sexual Sessions

Sexual acts do not occur at random across space and time. We have termed the primary chunk of sexual behaviour the sexual session or sexual encounter. A session consists of an ordered set of sexual acts involving one or more people in a specific place over a relatively short time. It is worth considering each of the elements of this definition in some detail.

Definitionally, sessions consist of one or more sexual acts, ordered either sequentially or simultaneously. While there are some acts which are physically impossible to do simultaneously, there is no logical reason why acts should occur in particular sequences or groups. Yet, as we shall see, there are distinct patterns of acts, and these are, we suggest, culturally informed. Turner (1984) has pointed out that the body is a prime site of social control, and it would be perverse not to see in the common sequence of wanking, sucking, fucking some echo of socialisation, replayed as increasing intimacy, or assertion/abrogation of self. We treat this subject in more detail below, when discussing the specifics of anal intercourse between men (see Chapter 11). In the same way as it is not always possible to distinguish one act from another, so is it often in practice not always easy to decide whether one or other act follows, overlaps with or is simultaneous with another. This, though logically inconvenient, is not a major problem.

The timing of a session is sometimes difficult to determine. Whereas in some cases the action begins, continues and comes to an end without interruption or pause, in many cases sessions will have longeurs, while the participant(s) rest, get (un)dressed, answer the 'phone, feed the cat or any of those things that were earlier forgotten. How long a pause has to be before one extended session becomes two distinct ones is a matter of little practical import: a logical nicety, which the pedantic will delight in exploring at length. For men, a common marker of the end of a session is orgasm, but while this is common it is not universal: sessions may end without orgasm while others may continue after it.

Though it may seem to be clear-cut, it turns out that the question of determining the number of participants in a sexual session is far from straightforward. Rather than consider the difference between a solo session and one involving two people as discrete entities, it is possible to think in terms of points on a continuum. This may seem odd, but consider the following. A person alone in a room, wanking and doing whatever else turns them on, will commonly fantasise, establishing in some cases an imaginary or remembered other as the focus for erotic excitement. Otherwise, photographs of individuals in states of undress or provocative dress might be employed as a concrete focus of erotic interest. Magazines which reproduce still photographs of sexual sessions, either of individuals or of two or moresomes, provide not only external focus but also a sequence, a sexual activity which the reader is invited to follow. Textual descriptions of sexual sessions, telephone lines which play pre-recorded verbal descriptions of sexual sessions, videos of people having sex, all provide not only a focus of erotic attention, but also guide it temporally, seeking to heighten arousal and interest over a period of time. The consumer will have differing degrees of control over the timing. In the telephone case this is largely outside his control, while videos and text allow choices to be made, boring bits skipped or particular parts to be lingered over, All these modes of enjoyment involve only one participant directly but others are involved vicariously, either unknowingly, as in the fantasy built round the builder, the biker or the pizza boy casually encountered during the day, or more directly, as when people are filmed having sex together.

In any meaningful sense of the term, however, it is clear that these scenarios involve only one participant. It is from this only a small step to consider an individual pleasuring him/herself in the presence of (an)other(s). These others might, indeed, be the photographers, filmers or spectators at a live sex show, in which case they themselves may or may not be sexually aroused, and the main participant may seek to dismiss their presence from their minds, as do some strippers who report thinking about the shopping to distance themselves from the scenario. In other cases the presence of the other can be a source of excitement. Having sex in public places can carry an extra erotic charge because of the reactions of unwitting others. In specifically defined erotic spaces, however, the presence of another may also be a source of narcissistic pleasure. It turns me on that he is turned on by me, even though I find him physically unattractive. Otherwise it is the derived pleasure of the other which is itself reflexively exciting. He turns me on; seeing him getting turned on turns me on and great sex can happen without physical contact. In these cases it makes sense to talk of two (or more) participants, even though physical contact may not be involved (such as on an interactive 'phone line).

The project makes a distinction between participants and sexual partners. A participant becomes a partner when physical contact is made (but see below). Clearly, this criterion describes not a discrete class of events but a continuum. Two men having sex in a cruising ground, for example, may be masturbating while watching each other. Physical contact might be non-existent, or confined to, say, the chest or the back and confined to friendly encouragement: a positive stroke. On the other hand, it might be specifically sexual and focused on particular areas, the nipples, the armpit, the toes, even the genitals, which give direct sexual charges. At this point participants merge into partners and may engage in any or all of the acts mentioned above.

A similar continuum can be constructed between twosomes and threesomes, ranging from the couple constructing a fantasy scenario, through watching a video and tempering their action to the development of that session, through the unwitting, witting, non-participation or involvement of another person. Further definitional complications arise in the case of threesomes if one person is excluded from the action for a time or if people wander into and out of the action.

The point is that sex is not simple. A comprehensive study of sex and sexuality should include aspects of all of these. Our primary interest in HIV transmission allowed us to concentrate on partners and to exclude from detailed consideration the complications of participation, erotic focus, intentionality and control that we have mentioned. Given that specific interest and the specific role played by anal and vaginal intercourse in the transmission of HIV, we also distinguished within the category partner, the category penetrative sexual partner (PSP), which was defined as: 'a sexual partner whom you fucked (either anally or vaginally) or who fucked you' (see Chapter 9 for the conceptual and epidemiological consequences of this).

It may come as a surprise, given the examples that we have adduced so far, but it is only at the level of the session that the sex and the gender of the participants become relevant. The fact that the participants are, for example, both female will exclude the possibility of an act involving the penis, and two men will not be able to have vaginal intercourse. Moreover, certain combinations of acts will not be possible in specific circumstances. A man and a woman will not be able to fuck each other (if we take fuck to involve the penis). Each session has a sexuality, derived from the sex of its participants. The issue of gender is altogether more complicated: although some people might think that, for example, a man dressed and acting as a woman would be constrained to 'feminine' roles, this is not the case.

Sexual Individuals

The sexual career of an individual can now be defined as the sum of the sessions in which s/he has participated. On this basis it is possible, at least in principle (in practice it is, as we shall see, fraught with problems), to distinguish completely homosexual and completely heterosexual individuals and to describe individuals with varying degrees of bisexual experience. This is not to restrict the sexual to the physical. We recognise that sexual behaviour and sexual interest or preference are both logically and empirically distinct. A sexual identity does not confine sexual practice, nor does sexual behaviour predict identification. There are clearly degrees of discordance: married men have sex with other men; gay men covertly have sex with women; and lesbians may have sex with men for pleasure or money. Many more will have fantasies at odds with their chosen identification. The relationship between avowed identity and behaviour is at best probabilistic.

Although sexual individuals are logically third-order constructs, they are the primary units of most studies of sexual behaviour. It is difficult to think of a method of sampling directly sexual sessions. The formulation above is intended to clarify the relationship between acts, sessions and individuals, a matter which we take up in more detail in the next section of this chapter.

We are now in a position to list the main counts of sexual behaviour used in the rest of this volume. Various statistics will be presented, referring to various time periods, the main ones being: whole life, last five years, last year and last month. For most of these time periods we may report the proportion of men who:

have at least one sexual partner;
have at least one PSP;
have engaged in each of the (modulated) sexual acts.

For those who fall into these categories, we may also report:

numbers of partners and PSPs;
number of times engaged in a particular act (only really feasible for shorter, more recent time periods).

Problems of Sampling

Whatever problems surround the definition of terms, the practical problem of selecting respondents for a study of male homosexual behaviour remains. Any sampling strategy is a compromise between the demands of the problem being addressed and the resources available for its solution, with the last word usually being reserved for the latter consideration. The purpose of sampling is to estimate the numerical characteristics of a population by directly examining only a subset of that population. Most commonly, sampling is random, in the sense that the probability of inclusion in the sample is the same (and greater than zero) for each member of the population. In this case a well known battery of statistical techniques is available to indicate the accuracy with which the sample statistics predict those of the population.

The question of defining the population from which such a sample might be drawn is, however, far from straightforward. Male homosexual behaviour is distributed throughout the male population, and not confined to that section which labels itself as 'gay'. This suggests that we investigate the incidence, range and frequency of homosexual behaviour in the whole of the male population. Indeed, in 1948 Kinsey wrote: 'Satisfactory incidence figures on the homosexual cannot be obtained by any technique short of a carefully planned population survey' (p. 618). During the last few years a national survey of sexual behaviour has been undertaken in Britain and is expected to publish its findings after this volume has gone to press. This survey will present figures for that portion of the male population which reports sex with men. With a sample size of some 20,000, such a project may be expected to render a definitive answer to the question, 'how many are there?' There are, however, good reasons to expect that the number reported by these methods will be an underestimate. As Cochran, Mosteller and Tukey (1954) point out in their exhaustive examination of the statistical procedures of Kinsey *et al.*, the problem is one of non-response.

> [N]o sex study of a broad human population can expect to present incidence data for reported behaviour that are known to be correct to within a few percentage points. Even with the best available sampling techniques,

> there will be a certain percentage of the population who refuse to give histories. If the percentage of refusals is 10% or more, then however large the sample, there are no statistical principles which guarantee that the results are correct to within two or three percent. . . . [A]ny claim that this is true must be based on the undocumented opinion that the behaviour of those who refuse to be interviewed is not very different from that of those who are interviewed. (p. 675)

In wave four (1991–92) of our work we explained the sampling strategy of the national survey and asked respondents whether they would be prepared to take part. Only about 50% said that they would not do so. Bearing in mind that our cohort may be presumed to overrepresent the most self-confident gay men, it must be concluded that the rate of refusal among those with homosexual experience who are less self-confident and assertive will be higher, and these rates of refusal are likely to be much higher than those reported as a whole for the national survey.

Added to this is the problem of non-response or obfuscation by those who do take part. As long as homosexual behaviour remains stigmatised, the presumption must be that there will be underreporting. Put bluntly, there are no good reasons for assuming that men who have not had homosexual experience will claim to have done so and every reason to believe that some men with such experience will disclaim it. If we add to this the problems admitted by Wellings *et al.* (1990) in finding a universally understood form of language, our conclusion must hold. The question of how much of an underestimate the figures will be is not answerable with any accuracy.

Sampling in Published Studies

Kinsey's own survey was a prodigious feat of data collection. He and his colleagues collected 12,000 life histories, of which the 5300 which refer to white males form the basis of the published work (1948: 6). The sampling technique used is cluster sampling (Cochran *et al.*, 1954: 689) in the sense that individuals were not drawn individually from the population but in groups. Kinsey described (1948: 13–16) the groups who provided help and data for the study including some fourteen colleges and universities which each provided more than 100 interviewees, the Kansas State Police, numerous hospitals and medical schools together with unsuspecting hitch hikers and train travellers cornered by the researchers.

The sampling procedures in studies concerned specifically with homosexuality vary from the opportunistic to the indefensible. Until the 1960s the populations studied were typically those imprisoned for their actions or undergoing treatment for their desires (Bergler, 1956; Bieber *et al.*, 1962, Schofield, 1965a). Such studies were criticised for generalising from the experience of the unfortunate few to the invisible majority, and in the late 1950s and 1960s descriptions of that wider homosexual society began to appear, either by 'self-confessed' homosexuals (Plummer, 1963; Cory, 1953; Cory and Leroy, 1963) or by concerned liberals (Magee, 1966; Chesser, 1959; Westwood, 1952, 1960; Hauser, 1962).

In the 1970s studies began to appear concerned with documenting the range and diversity of gay experience as the community emerged from the closet.

Typically if not exclusively written from within the gay community itself, these were remarkable for the positive attitude towards gay sexuality and experience that they displayed.

Harry (1976) and Harry and DeVall (1978: 23–7) surveyed 243 men from three sources in Detroit. They distributed questionnaires through two bartenders working in eight bars in the city, who were 'instructed to select persons from a wide variety of ages, life-styles and occupational background' (p. 24); through a 'distinguished older professional', who gave access to more covert social circles; and through three homophile organisations in the area. Saghir and Robins (1973) recruited eighty-nine gay men from homophile organisations in Chicago and San Francisco. Blumstein and Schwartz (1976) interviewed seventy-five ambisexual men. Schafer (1977) used 581 West German males. Jay and Young (1979), Spada (1979) and Barrington (1981), whose aim, it is probably fair to say, was as prurient as it was scientific, used the responses from questionnaires published in the gay press to present their data on the sexual experience of gay men.

From about the same time, various studies have documented the ethnography of homosexual interaction, beginning with the classic account by Humphreys (1970) of 'tearoom' sex, which the British prefer to term 'cottaging' (see Chapter 10). These include the cruising area (Delph, 1978; Harris, 1973; Seabrook, 1976: 117–19), the highway pick-up area (Corzine and Kirby, 1977), the intriguing 'homosexual drive-in' (Ponte, 1974) and the baths or saunas (Styles, 1979; Rumaker, 1978). Such studies are invaluable in illuminating the lifestyles of some and the fantasies of many more, but none is concerned to estimate the popularity of the pursuit.

In an important article Martin Weinberg (1970) suggests using samples drawn from a range of sites in order to maximise the range of experience covered. This approach has been favoured by Weinberg and his collaborators and has met with some success. Weinberg and Williams (1974; also Hammersmith and Weinberg, 1973) describe a three-nation, comparative survey. A total of 1057 questionnaires were distributed to individuals in the USA, drawn from mailing lists, club members and 'every seventh person in a random sample of 25 homosexual bars in San Francisco . . . [and] 20 [bars] in Manhattan' (p. 122). A total of 1077 respondents were found in Amsterdam using mailing lists and from those attending clubs and bars, and the same strategy in Denmark produced 303 replies (p. 123). They report that their respondents were skewed towards the higher educated and those in higher social classes, and tended to live in the larger cities.

Probably the most thorough sampling strategy in a study before 1980 is that of Bell and Weinberg (1978) in their major Kinsey Institute study. They used a number of different strategies to recruit potential respondents to a pool, from which pool the eventual interviewees were chosen (pp. 29–40). They made use of (1) advertisements and features in the press, (2) visits to bars and bath-houses, (3) personal contacts of those already recruited, (4) memberships of gay organisations and (5) the frequenters of 'public places' (for which read cruising grounds). The selection of the eventual respondents was made by means of what the authors call a stratified random sample from that pool (p. 34). This is misleading. The randomness of this procedure in no way guarantees the representativeness of the pool from which they were drawn, only that those selected are representative of those in the pool. Thus the procedure they describe would be more accurately labelled a quota sample.

If there is a major criticism of Bell and Weinberg's strategy, it is that the sampling procedures do not take full account of the existence of homosexual men who are not involved 'on the scene': a variant of the non-response problem discussed by Cochran *et al.* (1954, see above). With the exception of their 'public places' recruiting (which generated 4% of the pool and 9% of the final sample), all their methods assume that homosexual men have some involvement in the gay life of San Francisco. It may be, of course, that the homosexual population of that city is all or mostly thus involved, but this must remain a matter of conjecture.

A Return to First Principles

Two general criteria govern the composition of the sample required by a particular problem (Galtung, 19867: 51). First, its composition must be such that it is possible to test substantive hypotheses on it; and second, it must be possible to test hypotheses of generalisation from it. In the familiar case of probability sampling, both these criteria are satisfied (assuming sufficient size) by the randomness of the sampling. In cases where random selection is impossible, however, it is necessary to substitute a form of purposive sampling, which allows the testing of substantive hypotheses but not the testing of hypotheses of generalisation. Because of this loss of ability to generalise from the sample to the population with known degrees of accuracy, the method is frowned upon by many statisticians but is widely used in social science where populations are, for one reason or another, often unenumerable.

Quota sampling is perhaps the most widely used of the purposive sampling strategies. In this case the heterogeneity of the sample and its representativeness are guaranteed, not by random selection but by choosing respondents from the cells of a cross-classification of a number of variables (usually two or three), which, between them, account for a large proportion of the variation in the dependent variable(s). This procedure ensures, if the classifying variables are well chosen, that the full range of variation in the population is included in the sample. The essential flaw in the procedure is that it remains impossible to estimate the proportions of the whole population who fall into each of the cells of the classification and thus to weight the results from the sample to reproduce the population parameters. In the ideal case the whole of the variation in the dependent variable(s) is accounted for by the spanning variables and the cell entries reduce to replications in a form of quasi-experimental design.

The spanning variables choosen by SIGMA were age and relationship status. Age may be categorised in any number of ways, of course, but as has been pointed out, the peculiar and particular circumstances of the passing and provisions of the 1967 Act provide convenient and compelling break points. Those under age 21 (in 1987–88) are breaking the law if and when they engage in homosexual activity, while those who were over 21 but under 40 have spent the whole of their sexual maturity under its dispensation, in the light of gay liberation. They were therefore presumed to experience and express their sexuality in ways which differ from their older brethren.

Bell and Weinberg's typology of gay lifestyles combines two criteria, relationship status and amount of regret. We prefer to separate these two scales and use only relationship type for reasons that will become clearer later. As stressed

Table 6.1. Sampling Typology

	Age groups		
Relationship	Under 21	21–39	Over 39
Monogamous	I	II	III
Open (at least one regular partner and others)	IV	V	VI
No regular partner	VII	VIII	IX

above, we also hypothesise that the type and incidence of sexual behaviour will differ depending on age group. We therefore define a three-by-three typology as the basis of a sampling scheme, as illustrated in Table 6.1. Unfortunately, the definition of this typology does not begin to exhaust the sampling problems that face the study. The criticism above has focused on the undesirability of restricting attention to the gay community or to those who would identify as homosexual in a study which seeks to investigate the full range and incidence of male homosexual behaviour. Our criticism applies, with stronger reason, to those methods which favour the more articulate, better educated middle-class gay man. The force of this criticism behoves us, therefore, to ensure that the less articulate, the secretive and the 'dysfunctional' will be found and included in the sample.

To Trace a Snowball

An attractive means of moving towards this goal is to use the technique of snowballing, or, more accurately, tracing sampling. The essential idea is that a small group of individuals, 'seeds', are chosen and included in the sample. This group provides information on their friends (or contacts) and these are also included in the sample. The process of contacting the friends of friends is continued until the whole of the network thus described has been contacted or the required number of individuals has been included.

The method is well suited to the investigation of covert and hidden populations, since it allows the possibility of burrowing into those areas. It is surprising that the technique has not been more widely used in studies of homosexuality. Kinsey (1948: 40) describes an embryonic form of snowballing, and Westwood (1960), in a report commissioned by the British Social Biology Council, contacted eighty-nine of his 127 men 'through friends who had already been interviewed' (p. 2). In neither case was an attempt made to estimate the sampling error of the procedure (unsurprisingly, since the estimation procedure did not exist) or to assess the differences between first and subsequent order contacts. As Westwood (1952: 201) rightly points out, there is no way of knowing whether the distribution of types in his sample reflects that in the population as a whole (although see his unsubstantiated and contradictory claim quoted at the beginning of the next chapter).

Warren (1974) and Harry and DeVall (1978) both use the social networks of initial contacts to gain access to the more private areas of the gay world. Bell and Weinberg also use the friends of people already contacted by their multiple sampling strategies to top up their sample (1978: 31). It is, of course, somewhat ironic to use this sampling method in a study of the spread of HIV, since the same equations that describe the development of a snowball sample also model the epidemic process. The process whereby a sample is identified by a process that traces or snowballs outward from a small starting group is formally identical to the process whereby an epidemic is spread by contagion or infection (see Bartholomew, 1982, Chs. 9 and 10, for an overview).

SIGMA Research Design

Project SIGMA is a prospective cohort study, which involves following changes in the behaviour of a group of men over a period of time. Cohort studies, such as this, allow individual changes to be monitored and typically show higher rates of change than studies which take separate samples at different points in time. The study is unique in the UK in that it does not recruit from GUM clinics. Clinic studies, though valuable, are less representative of gay and bisexual men, because some men do not attend clinics and others may not admit to homosexual activity when they do.

The initial recruitment to the cohort occurred between September 1987 and August 1988, across ten cities in England and Wales. This we refer to as wave one. Four methods were used: following up respondents to an earlier postal questionnaire; leafleting social and commercial outlets; fulfilling speaking engagements; and following up contacts provided by other recruits.

> In 1984/85 a postal survey appeared in *Gay Times*, a national monthly gay news magazine, and *Capital Gay*, a weekly London oriented gay paper. Respondents to that survey who indicated a willingness to take part in the main project were contacted and invited to face-to-face interviews.
> Good relations were established with many social and commercial venues (pubs, clubs, social centres, etc.) and permission was gained for leafleting of these venues. The leaflets explained the nature and purpose of the research, while stressing confidentiality and the benefits to all of more being known about the spread of HIV infection.
> The principal investigators were all well known within gay social, political, counselling and befriending circles. Many of the research staff also had experience with one or more gay organizations. Opportunities were sought for all staff to address groups on the aims of the project and to seek volunteers.
> Each recruit was asked if they had friends or acquaintances who might wish to take part in the survey. This form of snowballing provided a means by which we might reach as far as possible into the population under investigation.

In the first wave 930 men were interviewed, of whom 310 were from London. All respondents originally recruited and interviewed in the first phase were recontacted. At each subsequent wave only those who had been interviewed in the previous wave were contacted again unless we had strong reasons to believe we could reconnect with a respondent (for example, if they had moved away but moved back again). However, funding restraints in the third phase meant that none of these could be reinterviewed at that time, although in the fourth phase all who were interviewed in the second phase were invited for interview. Since there were nearly two years between contacting this group it was unlikely to be particularly successful.

Respondents were recontacted three times: for wave two interviews between July 1988 and August 1989; again for wave three between September 1989 and June 1990, and for wave four between January 1991 and March 1992. The average (median) time between interviews was ten months. The total numbers interviewed at subsequent waves were 754, 374 and 472. The low recall figures in wave three (and hence wave four) were caused by funding only to reinterview in the two main sites. Because of the emphasis on two main sites in wave three, the proportion of men from London has risen from a third to just over a half; 274 men were interviewed in all four waves, and 358 were interviewed in wave one and again in wave four. Recontacting was always carried out on a strict basis, starting with those interviewed first at the previous phase, though when they were actually reinterviewed was dependent on the respondent himself. The bulk of the interviewing in each phase was carried out in an intense period of eight to ten months with a few earlier pilot interviews and a few stragglers later.

We always recognized that there might be greater difficulties in recruiting appropriate numbers of young, older and black/Asian gay men. Consequently special effort was made to reach such men. Although some success was achieved with older men in some sites and young men in others, results with minority ethnic groups were disappointing.

As noted earlier, the period of recruitment coincided with the promotion of Section 28 of the 1988 Local Government Act which was widely regarded as a thinly disguised denigration to second-class citizenship of non-heterosexuals. Consequently, this research, being funded by the government, was often regarded with suspicion.

The project was notified of eighteen deaths during the study, at least half of which were caused by illnesses related to HIV disease.

Multi-Centre: Why the Sites Were Chosen

When the proposal was being submitted for consideration, some evidence was emerging to indicate that (other factors being equal) attitudes held by and sexual behaviour patterns exhibited by gay and bisexual men in London were different from those held and exhibited in other parts of the country. To examine these and related matters appropriately, sites for investigation were chosen and quotas established for those to be sought for interview based on age and relationship type.

In London, a site of in-migration for gay men and lesbians, there are many diverse commercially-based social venues which cater specifically for gay men. There is also a large number of formally organized gay social and campaigning organisations and several voluntary charitable counselling and befriending organisations which specialise in calls from gay men. London is also a noted 'cosmopolitan area' and is known to be a place in which one may lose oneself. The London base for the research was within South Bank Polytechnic, more recently renamed South Bank University.

South Wales has a much smaller gay men's social scene, and much less open attitudes to same-sex activity and relationships prevail. Cardiff provides a focus for such commercial, social, campaigning, befriending and counselling activity as exists. Outside Cardiff, and to a lesser extent Swansea, the valley communities are often insular and there are very few places for gay men to meet except their own friendship networks, cruising areas and cottages. The Cardiff base for the research was within University College, Cardiff (later renamed the University of Wales College at Cardiff).

The researchers employed on this and related studies were, with one exception, based either in London or in Cardiff. The one exception was based within Newcastle-upon-Tyne Polytechnic. The gay men's social scene in the north-east of England is centred on Newcastle-upon-Tyne and to a lesser extent Teesside. Like South Wales, less open attitudes to same-sex activity and relationships prevail, and within the (former) mining communities there are few places for gay men to meet. Like Cardiff, Newcastle contained several commercial outlets and some social, campaigning, counselling and befriending activity.

Six other sites were nominated for study, all of them in England. (Funding to extend the project into Scotland was refused by the Scottish Office: AIDS was not, they commented, a problem among gay men in Scotland.) These sites were chosen to provide for a variety of region, size, the nature of gay men's social scene, and such attributes as nature of major employment in the area. The sites chosen were Birmingham, Bristol and Liverpool (administered from Cardiff); Portsmouth, Norwich and Leeds (administered from London); and Teesside (administered from Newcastle-upon-Tyne).

Dates of initial recruitment varied slightly between sites depending on factors such as availability of staff, staff training, accessibility of staff to site and points of contact for recruitment within the chosen site. Recruitment began first in London, Cardiff and Newcastle and only later in the seven subsidiary sites.

Sampling Strategy of the Project: Intention and Actuality

The original intention of the project was to select cities within which a range of gay venues could be targeted as sources for a starting sample. From these, a snowballing process would take place which would aim to fill the cells of the design. Two strategies were proposed to do this — either (1) a type I person should nominate other type I people or (2) simply snowball. In practice, strategy (1) proved quite impractical and strategy (2) moderately successful. Overall, snowballing provided about a third of the eventual sample, though it never generated the bulk of the respondents as early plans had foreseen. The reasons for this were: (i) men were wary about giving names of friends, etc. without first asking permission; (ii) when they themselves volunteered to contact friends, chasing up was difficult and the response rate was low. The process, though it worked, worked very slowly and then fitfully and was a significant drain on resources. It was more cost-effective to concentrate on establishing first-order contacts rather than following up leads.

More emphasis was therefore placed on the first-order contacts. The main plan was to use respondents volunteering their names in a postal questionnaire circulated in the gay press in 1984/85 (a report of which appears in McManus and McEvoy, 1987) and to recruit from gay venues. This was obviously easier in

London, where there are more to choose from, and relatively easy in the cities where small samples were required — you are chasing a fairly low compliance rate. In Cardiff, on the other hand, the problem is greater, in that the required sample is a relatively large percentage of the gay population. Moreover, the researchers, being gay in the main and involved in the scene, faced problems and advantages. The advantage is that friends can be suborned, but the disadvantage is that there will always be people who are hostile and will refuse and, as happened, dissuade others from taking part in the study. The question we have to ask is whether this pattern of differential response affects the sexual behaviour data; that is, do those who did not take part have different patterns of sexual behaviour than those that do. The question is that of non-response mentioned earlier and is unanswerable in principle.

Asking Questions, Finding Answers

The Theoretical: The Problem of Knowledge

This book describes, primarily, the sexual behaviour of men. Such a bold statement, for all its simplicity, is, however, far from being unambiguous. As we have seen, the description of sexual behaviour soon becomes complex, and, as we shall see, an accurate account of those aspects of sexual behaviour which are relevant to our purpose is far from being an account of the totality of sexual behaviour. These accounts exist in the form of completed questionnaires and diary forms — written renditions of remembered activities constructed some time after the events described — at least in most cases. These accounts have been transferred from the written pages to computer files where various symbolic manipulations have been performed. Finally, these results, in the form of tables, figures and text, have been prepared and the physical result of this process is now in your hands.

Put rather differently, the process looks something like this. In January 1988, say, two men somewhere in the UK have sex together. Some time later one of them writes down a description of that encounter or provides an interview with some details, selecting those aspects which others — Project SIGMA — have deemed to be relevant. Some time later this description, together with others describing other sexual encounters, appears in an office in Cardiff or London, where, some time later, it is copied and edited into a computer file. Some time later this description, along with others provided by other individuals, is scanned by another person, who notes certain features of the records the frequency of this, the frequency of co-occurrence of this and that, and so on. Some time later again another person looks at the collection of such features as has been constructed, and from them fashions an account, called 'a book', which purports to be a description of sexual behaviour, and the question naturally arises: what is the relationship between this thing called 'book' and the thing called 'sexual behaviour'?

It is worth noting that both preceding descriptions are couched in the form of narratives, that is, sequences of actions which follow one another temporally and which are also presumed to be, in some sense, logically consequent upon one another. At each stage of the process we have described, the research process, someone seeks to construct a narrative (or at least a coherent account) of certain events.

1 The researchers decide:
  a) what is to be asked
  b) who is to be allowed to answer
  c) what counts as an acceptable response
2 The respondents decide:
  a) whether to answer these questions or not
  b) which aspects of his experience are relevant
  c) how to present/reconstruct these relevant experiences
3 The researchers decide:
  a) how much of this reconstruction to record
  b) in what form
4 The researchers decide:
  a) how to treat these records
  b) how to 'analyse' these records
5 The researchers decide:
  a) how to 'interpret' these analyses
  b) how to present these interpretations

At each stage, therefore, *relevance* is *negotiated.*

Such an account should make it clear that the notion that this research is value-free is untenable. Each negotiation, each decision about relevance, is made in a concrete political and social situation: the researchers decide what it is politically acceptable to research in negotiation with the funding bodies, the target population and academic peers: the researchee decides what is acceptable to admit to or boast about. Researchers decide what questions to ask of the data, which cross-tabulation or regression to perform in the light of their theories about the world, and then which of these results to emphasise and which to highlight in an account which, again, is prepared in a particular political context and social climate.

How much credence should be placed in the findings, and what is the relationship between the findings set out in this book and the 'truth'? Such questions inevitably arise and are, of their nature, unfortunately unanswerable. Three criteria might be used, however, in the attempt: technical competence, explicitness and relevance.

The techniques of survey research, in the broadest terms, figure in many an undergraduate syllabus, and our work, like any of its kind, may be judged in terms of its technical competence: are the methods employed appropriate and properly applied? There are three positions, however, from which we would distance ourselves. First, we would not claim, as an unreconstructed positivist might, that the proper application of the methods of scientific enquiry automatically lead to the 'truth'. There have been, in the past, some criticisms of our work which have, explicitly or implicitly, assumed that we hold that view. We hope that the content of this book makes it clear that we are not so naive. Second, we refuse to accept that the use of quantitative methods automatically commits us to a dehumanising, cold-blooded view of human behaviour, which exalts quantification over the lived experience of individuals.

There remains a third criticism, which we hear all too often. Few things are more irritating than the smug smile on the face of a questioner who has forced the admission that the sample is non-random, and therefore unrepresentative. As s/he sits back, convinced that the entire study can be dismissed out of hand for this reason, it is easy to wonder not only at the smugness but at the naivete of supposing that, in the eight years or so that the study has been discussed and executed, the problem of representativeness had not arisen. We ask not to be absolved from criticism: there are many flaws in the execution of the project which hindsight unerringly identifies. We ask only to be judged against a criterion of practical rather than idealistic competence.

This brings us to the second major criterion: explicitness. It is a feature of the sort of work we have undertaken that the process be open to inspection and criticism. We ask to be judged on the process of arriving at conclusions as well as their content. This can be both a weakness and a strength. It is a weakness in that it opens up a host of possibilities of criticism, which critical theorists, whose pronouncements are judged only at the altar of political correctness and expediency, do not have to face. It is, however, simultaneously a strength, in that, if the method can be shown to be sound, the conclusions, however unpalatable or inconvenient, must be afforded some respect. Our duty, therefore, is to conduct the research as well as possible and to set out the process of reaching conclusions as clearly as possible. Whether we have succeeded in this, it is not for us to say.

This brings us to the third major criterion: relevance. As can be seen from the discussion above, while relevance is negotiated by both researchers and respondents, the former are in a much stronger position of power. Not only do they initially set the agenda and at more points in the research process determine how to treat the data; they also have the ability to censor the respondent. This can be done either by intention or by accident. In both cases relevant information may be lost, but is must be borne in mind that decisions in the research process *must* be made. It is not possible to gather all the minutiae about an individual's sexual behaviour and lifestyle, and look at them in the context of a host of other people's details. This is not possible for a number of reasons, not least of which is, as we have seen, what counts as 'sexual behaviour' is infinitely variable. In practice, what is relevant to the questions in hand must be determined, and while the respondent must have a say in this, it is ultimately the researcher who must make the decision. If it is left solely to respondents, in all likelihood one would end with as many relevance criteria as one has respondents.

What the researchers decide is relevant to their enterprise will in all likelihood change over the course of a long-term project such as SIGMA. Some things will fade from view as their utility to understanding diminishes, other aspects of people's lives will gain in prominence as new insights are developed. At the final count it is the task of others to determine the relevance of the work to the issues it set out to address. No project can claim to cover all aspects of people's lives. However, where sexual behaviour is concerned, claims can be made that the most relevant aspects, that is those aspects of people's lives that have the greatest bearing on their sexual behaviour, have been covered. It is only in comparison with other research projects that these claims can be accepted or rejected.

The Practical

In a project stretching over a period of years and involving four waves of data collection as well as numerous other information collecting exercises, it is inevitable that ideas about what is and is not relevant information will change, both as contemporary concerns about HIV change and as the information base of the project itself expands. Thus, for example, in the first phase of the project the emphasis was still on the uptake of safer sex practices, whereas in the latest phase the compelling debates have been around the notion of 'relapse'. Similarly, in an attempt to situate the information coming from the project in as wide a social context as possible, the first question schedule included questions on first sexual experience, social class background and other general questions, which, once asked, need not be repeated.

The project has, in each of its data collection phases, interviewed all respondents face-to-face, who were:

asked in detail about their sexual histories and current sexual behaviour; their knowledge, attitudes and beliefs about AIDS/HIV and safer sex and a variety of other matters;
asked to reconstruct in detail a sexual diary for the preceding week, noting the time and place of each sexual session, the partner(s) involved (if any) and the exact sequence of sexual acts, together with the use of toys, accompaniments, etc. and noting the use of condoms in particular;
asked to keep a diary of their sexual activity for the month following interview (about 20–30% do so in each wave);
asked but not required to give a sample of blood or saliva for testing for HIV antibodies. Pre-test counseling was given, and results of blood tests were available if requested. When results were given to respondents, post-test counselling was also supplied.

The Questionnaire

The questionnaire or structured interview has been at the heart of sexual research since the earliest days (Hirschfeld, 1920). Their use reaches its zenith in Kinsey's work, and his discussion of the matter (1948: 35ff.) remains exemplary. Interviews and/or self-completion questionnaires were used by many of his successors and imitators, especially in the 1970s (Bell and Weinberg, 1978; Spada, 1979; Jay and Young, 1979). By this time, however, the use of questionnaires and interviews had come under sustained attack as the ethnomethodological critique challenged the epistemological, methodological and technical bases of positivist science, and the central texts of the contemporary gay movement, especially Plummer's (1975) are openly hostile to positivism and its methods, as we have outlined in Chapter 1.

At the heart of this debate lies the question of objectivity. In the crudest terms, positivism asserts the possibility of objective knowledge, which is attainable through the application of scientific methods. These methods, if correctly applied, guarantee to unearth the 'truth' and they are qualitatively distinct from everyday processes of human problem-solving. The critique of this approach asserts, by contrast, that objective knowledge is unattainable. Scientific method, in this account, is one among many ways of constructing knowledge, but it gives no automatic access to truth and is not qualitatively distinct from the means by which ordinary people construct everyday knowledge. Their approach therefore centres on the process of *verstehen*, an attempt to understand social processes as they are understood by the people involved.

The debate is now an old one and is rehearsed with dispiriting frequency in any number of undergraduate essays. This is not the place to rehearse the intricacies or the history of that debate, except to point out that it continues to reverberate in HIV research. Most behavioural research carried out in the USA and contained in the scientific journals adheres, often uncritically, to the positivist methodology, with its concentration on quantification and its apparatus of hypothesis testing. On the other hand, anthropologists have been vociferous in asserting the utility of methods focused on meanings (for a review and extensive bibliography see Herdt *et al.*, 1991). Yet others, including ourselves, have espoused a pragmatic approach, which seeks to side-step the philosophical debate and to deploy methods which are appropriate to answering different questions.

The project decided to use a structured interview schedule as the main means of obtaining data. The question which needs to be answered regards the appropriateness of this method to the questions which Project SIGMA sought to ask. The structured interview is generally criticised on three main grounds. First, it imposes the researcher's frame of reference on the respondent. Since the researcher controls not only the content but also the form and the order of the questions asked, critics claim that the respondent is herded into answering the questions in the way that the researcher expects, rather than expressing his or her 'real' feelings, ideas and attitudes. Feminist methodology has done much to further this view. Second, and related to the first point, structured interviews are thought to create a distance and a power imbalance between the (powerful) interviewer and the (powerless) respondent.By taking control of the interaction, the researcher is accused of browbeating the respondent and alienating them from their authentic experience. Third, and again leading from this, it is said that the structured interview, by its form, restricts attention to that which can be quantified and is relatively poor at exploring the complexity of individual response.

At base, therefore, the structured interview approach maximises reliability while being of more dubious validity. The other approach strives for validity, but in the process sacrifices reliability and comparability. The original focus of the project, certainly as far as the funding authorities were concerned, was the provision of estimates of sexual practices that would inform epidemiological modelling and also rational bases for the planning of future services. We were, therefore, committed to a large-scale, quantitative study by the very nature of our research question. Questionnaires and structured interviews remain one of the most useful, perhaps the only, feasible means of gathering large amounts of data from large numbers of people. The choice lay between these two methods. Given the need to maximise validity, the need to collect serum samples (see below) and the sensitive nature of the subject matter, a structured interview was preferred.

At each wave of the project a questionnaire was designed, which sought to combine comparability with earlier waves, and other projects in other countries with emergent concerns and background data. The length of the questionnaire decreased over the waves. Wave one ran to three and a half hours on average, wave four to about an hour. This was due mainly to the need to collect data in the earlier waves on background, history and personal details which needed not be repeated.

The content of the first wave schedule was as follows:

Personal information including: age, occupation, relationship status, home background, involvement in gay community, political and religious beliefs

Sexual orientations (activities and feelings)
Disclosure of homosexuality
(Regular) sexual relationships
Coming out: biographical data

Numbers and characteristics of sexual partners
Sexual behaviour inventory
Retrospective weekly sexual diary
Attitudes to and feelings about sexual acts

General health
HIV testing
Disclosure of HIV status (where relevant)
Use of medical services, STD history
Safer sex knowledge and attitudes
Knowledge about AIDS, people with AIDS, etc.
Social activities and non-sexual lifestyle
Drug and alcohol use

Such detailed questions about intimate and private behaviour require a significant degree of trust and rapport between interviewer and respondent. Although we maximised cooperation by methodological, strategic and other means outlined here and elsewhere (Coxon *et al.*, 1993), we are very aware that there is a strong relativity here: within a marginalised or socially invisible group the same issues arise as in the general population — there are still sensitive areas (but different ones) which require much the same techniques to overcome. Thus, following the lead of Kinsey (1948) and Schofield (1965a), we used a question format that aimed to give respondents permission to discuss all the aspects of their sexual behaviour. We asked, 'When did you last . . .?', thereby implying we assumed they (and thus all those we interviewed) engaged in the activity involved. This, we assume, overcomes some of the problems of estimating the prevalence and incidence of activities which many (including some gay men) would find problematic.

However, the success of this strategy still depends on skilled interviewers establishing rapport and permission to talk. With regard to interviewers, respondents were able to nominate (or refuse) a given interviewer, either by name or in terms of their gender and/or sexual orientation. Although most research staff were gay or bisexual, we have employed and used heterosexual and lesbian women and heterosexual men. Interviewer recruitment, selection and training were rigorous, and involved regular monitoring, supervision and deselection where necessary.

It was relatively simple to arrange for interviewers to be trained in counselling, though it was a novelty for research staff to be told that such training and the taking of blood was part of their conditions of appointment. Arrangements

Table 6.2. Scientific Terms and Most Common Preferred Terms for Fourteen Core Sexual Activities

Scientific name	Preferred terms
Masturbation	Wanking
Fellation	Sucking
Anal intercourse	Fucking
Anodigital insertion	Fingering
Anilingus	Rimming
Deep kissing	Kissing
Frottage	Body rubbing
Massage	Massage
Inter-femoral intercourse	Thigh-fucking
Corporal punishment	CP/Spanking
Lindinism/urolagnia	Water sports
Anobrachial intercourse	Fisting
Enemas	Douching
Coprophilia	Scat

had also to be made for communicating the test results, and for safeguarding the data about a subject's serostatus. The act of taking blood established a quite distinctive — and sometimes almost proprietorial — bond between the interviewer and respondent. This could certainly increase rapport, but it also introduced interesting examples of role conflict (Coxon *et al.*, 1993).

It became apparent that despite general willingness (and even enthusiasm) for respondents to share a good deal of intimate detail with the interviewer, there were certain areas of sensitivity, 'shading' and even downright lying in the interview. These areas usually included marginalised sexual behaviour (e.g., anobrachial intercourse, or fisting). Less expectedly, it also turned out that probably the most sensitive issue of all was sex for money (in either direction). This we discovered primarily by a debriefing procedure where we colluded in lying by saying, 'Well, we know people sometimes lie about some things in the interview . . . would you like to say where you did?'

The sexual terminology used during interviews was within the control of individual respondents. They were asked to indicate their preferred term for each sexual act, and these terms were used for the rest of the interview/s. Presented on the right of Table 6.2 are the most common preferred terms. Street terms were preferred by the vast majority of men.

Bleeding

A description of the methods used to take and test samples of blood and saliva will be found in Chapter 8.

Confidentiality

Confidentiality of data is always a problem in social science research. It becomes doubly sensitive when the behaviour concerned is proscribed and/or illegal, and where the sexual orientation of the subject might be a closely guarded secret. The problems are aggravated when the study is longitudinal, since the identity of each respondent is needed for tracking purposes. When, as here, the question of HIV serostatus is added, the problems are further aggravated, especially in a climate where anti-gay and anti-people with HIV legislation is being enacted.

Respondents in Project SIGMA were promised confidentiality in that their names and addresses would be kept under strict security and not linked to data at any time. The link between the project code number and name and address was made only at the time of interview. Respondents were also guaranteed anonymity for anyone they chose to mention during the course of the interview, and were encouraged to use acronyms or first names, most particularly when they referred to sexual partners. Respondents were by and large more concerned about protecting the identity of their friends and nominees than protecting their own.

Further details of the mechanisms employed by the project in the course of data collection will be found in Coxon *et al.* (1993).

Notes

1 An important part of the project's data collection methods was the use of diaries for analysis of the details of sexual behaviour. This method is described in Coxon (1988), Davies and Coxon (1990) and Coxon *et al.* (1992). Further discussion is omitted from this volume since it does not make use of the diary data.

2 The gendering of sexual language and its rendition in terms of activity and passivity is pervasive. It does not seem to be possible, without absurdly long periphrases, to avoid this. The terms are, therefore, rendered in nonce marks.

7 Demographic Description

> The research worker is able to state with some confidence, from all that he has learned during the course of this two-year research, that every type of man who admits he is homosexual is included in this sample. (Westwood, 1952: 201)

Any study which looks at the some aspects of the lives of a large number of people must make some assessment of other characteristics of that population. This is in order to gauge how homogeneous the population is in terms of important social variables such as age, education, social class, etc. While we make no such grandiose claims as Westwood, in this chapter we present details of the social background of the cohort at first interview, then discuss data reliability and attrition across all sites.

Wave One Demographics

Age

The age distribution is given in Table 7.1. Notable overall features are:

the median age was 29, with a range from 15 to 81 years;
111 respondents were under 21, the age of consent;
349 respondents were 25 or younger.

Given the sampling strategy, it is not possible to say whether this distribution reflects the actual age profile of the gay population. The overrepresentation in the 21–40 range almost certainly reflects the influence of gay liberation (see Chapter 6).

Marital Status

Marital status is shown in Table 7.2. In short,

4% are currently married and a further 8% were separated, divorced or widowed.

Table 7.1. Age Distribution

Statistics	All	London	Outside London
Median	29	30	28
Upper quartile	38	39	37
Lower quartile	23	25	22
Range	15–81	16–81	15–76
Mean	32.0	33.8	31.2
Age groups			
Under 21	111	23	88
21 to 29	369	126	243
30 to 39	258	85	173
40 and over	192	76	116
Total	930	310	620

Table 7.2. Marital Status

Percentage	Married[1]	Single	SWD[2]
London	3.5	87.7	7.8
Outside London	4.2	87.0	7.8
Total	4.0	87.2	7.8

Notes: [1] Includes current cohabitation with a woman.
[2] Separated, Widowed or Divorced.

Table 7.3. Highest Educational Qualifications

Percentage	O level or less	A level or equivalent	Degree or more
London	24.0	29.5	46.4
Outside London	37.7	34.2	28.1
Total	33.2	32.6	34.2

While it is not possible to say whether this is a representative proportion of gay married men, the prevalence is very close to that found by other researchers (Connell *et al.*, 1988; Ross, 1990).

Educational Qualifications

Respondents were asked what educational qualifications they held. Highest educational qualifications (HEQ) are shown in Table 7.3. Tabulations of HEQ sharply differentiate the sample from the wider population and yield notable differences between London and other sites. The first of these may be related to the nature of the study, the type of recruitment and the environments in which researchers usually mix. However, it may also be related to the characteristics of the underlying population, in that those with more formal education may be better able to cope with any conflict they feel between their feelings and hostility within society towards same-sex relationships.

The difference between London and other sites may be explicable by a phenomenon much commented on in the gay press, that of higher educated young gay men being able to move from provincial towns to London to escape perceived social pressures and to create their own social environment. Outside London those with qualifications less than A levels form between 32.6% (Liverpool+) and 40.1% (Newcastle+), and those with degree qualifications form between 24.1% (Newcastle+) and 31.1% (Liverpool+); in both cases London is notably outside the range.

About a third (33%) had O level qualifications or less;
Another third (34%) had a degree or equivalent.

Social Class

Social class was determined by allocating reported occupation to the social class categories of the registrar general's classification. In summary:

half of the respondents were in social classes 1 and 2 (managerial, professional or non manual);
just over a third were in social class categories 3, 4 and 5;
a sixth were unemployed, students or retired.

It is clear that the cohort is more educated and belongs to a higher social class than the population as a whole. This undoubtedly reflects the greater willingness of men in these groups to take part in studies such as this. The same overrepresentation is commonly found in such studies (see, for example, Connell *et al.*, 1988).

Sexual Preference

Respondents were asked to use the Kinsey scale (below) to indicate how they rated themselves both in terms of their sexual feelings and their sexual activity.

0 exclusively heterosexual
1 mainly heterosexual but with a small degree of homosexuality
2 mainly heterosexual but with a substantial degree of homosexuality
3 equally heterosexual and homosexual
4 mainly homosexual but with a substantial degree of heterosexuality
5 mainly homosexual but with a small degree of heterosexuality
6 exclusively homosexual

These results are summarised in Table 7.4.

Between London and other sites there is very little variability.
The majority classified themselves as exclusively or predominantly homosexual in terms of both feelings (93%) and activity (95%).

Table 7.4. Percentages Reporting Kinsey Ratings 3 to 6

Activity	3	4	5	6
% London	0.3	2.3	14.4	83.0
% Outside London	2.4	3.4	15.4	78.8
% Total	1.7	3.0	15.1	80.2
Feelings	3	4	5	6
% London	2.9	2.3	29.3	65.5
% Outside London	3.5	4.0	31.8	60.7
% Total	3.3	3.4	31.0	62.3

Sexual Preference and Sexual Activity

While there is a high correlation between the scales of feeling and activity (68.3% give the same answer to both questions), the fit is not perfect. Not only do some of the few self-identified bisexuals only have sex with men (or even less commonly only with women) but almost 5% of the men who see themselves as predominantly or exclusively homosexual (Kinsey scale 5s and 6s) have sex with women.

> Thus homosexual activity, or even a gay identity, do not foreclose on heterosexual behaviour: that is, 12% were behaviourally bisexual (sex with men and women in last year).

Sexual Identity

> The overwhelming majority of respondents chose to call themselves gay.

Disclosure

It was an integral part of the sampling strategy to seek to include in the cohort men who had not disclosed their sexuality to significant others.

> Under a quarter (22%) were out as gay to all their family, friends and workmates.
> Just under a third (32%) were out to fewer than half to these.

Self-Acceptance

Respondents were asked whether they regretted being gay. Table 7.5 shows the results.

> Two-thirds (66%) indicated no regret at being gay.
> Less than a quarter (21%) indicated a little regret.

Table 7.5. Percentages Reporting Degrees of Regret at Being Homosexual

Percentage	London	Outside London	All
None	68.1	65.3	66.3
A little	21.1	21.5	21.4
Somewhat	9.7	10.9	10.5
Great deal	1.0	2.3	1.8

Note: Figures refer only to those rating 3–6 on the Kinsey feelings scale.

Two other related questions were asked: 'If there were a pill that would make you completely and permanently heterosexual would you take such a pill today?'

> Less than a tenth (9%) would take a pill today to make then heterosexual.

However, rather wider differences between London and other cities emerged when another question on this theme were asked, namely: 'Have you ever seriously considered discontinuing your homosexual activity?'

> Less than a fifth (17%) had considered giving up sexual activity with other men.

In this case, however, in London only 5.5% said 'yes' whereas it was 23.1% elsewhere.

On all these counts, however, our sample seem to be more self-accepting and comfortable with being gay than those in the sample studied by Bell and Weinberg (1978). In their study 27% regretted being gay, 29% had seriously considered giving up being gay, and 14% said they would take a pill to make them heterosexual. The difference in results may be explained by recruitment methods, cultural differences between US and UK, or changes in social climate which make it easier for some to accept their sexuality in the late 1980s than at the end of the 1970s. As likely as any of these reasons is, however, what must not be ignored was the desire of the respondent to present himself as self-accepting to an interviewer who (almost without exception) was self-identified as gay and could have been presumed to be self-accepting.

Ethnic Origin

Despite serious efforts, attempts to secure a group of black respondents large and diverse enough for meaningful comparisons to be made were not successful.

> Just under 5% of the cohort were from black and ethnic minority populations.

Table 7.6. Political Affiliation (percentages)

Percentage	Labour	Conservative	Liberal/SDP	Other*
London	49.4	13.9	14.8	21.9
Outside London	46.9	16.0	14.5	22.6
Total	47.7	15.3	14.6	22.4

Note: * Other includes those who expressed support for other parties, those who stated they had sympathy with no party, and those who refused to answer.

Political Affiliation

Respondents were asked: 'With which political party are you most in sympathy?' The interviews encompassed the period in which the alliance between the Liberal Party and the Social Democratic Party was being transformed into a combined Social and Liberal Democratic Party and a separate Social Democratic Party. The period pre-dates rise and fall in support for the Green Party, and the reformation of the Liberal Democratic and Social Democratic parties into the Social and Liberal Democrats.

The results presented in Table 7.6 cannot be seen as a political opinion polling exercise. However, the results are consistent across administrative jurisdiction and do differ sharply from those of polling exercises during the period of interview in showing rather more support for the Labour Party and rather less for the Conservative Party than in the electorate at large.

Religious Affiliation

Respondents were also asked: 'How religious would you say you are?' and given six options: very religious indeed; very religious; quite religious; not at all religious; not at all religious (agnostic); not at all religious (atheist). They were then asked: 'Which religious or humanist organization do you belong to?' Only 12.2% of respondents claimed allegiance to one of two major Christian denominations, (8.2% Anglican and 4.0% Roman Catholic), with no difference between London and elsewhere, and a further 4.5% claimed allegiance to other religious or humanist bodies.

Data Reliability

Without a denominator study, it is, impossible to assess exactly how representative such a cohort is (Davies, 1986), just as it is impossible to judge the representativeness of clinic-based studies. However, this study remains the largest ever undertaken in the UK, and the diversity of the recruitment sources gives grounds for believing the data are robust. Also, it may be reasonably assumed that the cohort includes a wider cross-section of the male homosexually active population, in terms of social and sexual activity, than those studies which recruit either exclusively or predominantly from clinics.

Questions regarding sexual behaviour and condom use refer to the month preceding interview. This is a shorter period than that used by Salzman *et al.* (1987), who used a test-retest procedure to establish that self-reported homosexual behaviour in interviews covering such short periods of time is a reliable method. In this cohort estimates of lifetime partner numbers from wave one were used in a test-retest procedure against lifetime partner numbers from wave two (minus the number of partners in last year). No significant difference was found between the two measures ($t = 0.607$, $p. = 0.54$).

Internal checks have also been carried out to confirm the reliability of the data. One test for reliability is to compare reported frequencies of insertive and receptive anal intercourse. If the data are reliable, then in a closed system the two estimates would be asymptotically equal. The alternative hypothesis that, given the stigma attached to receptive anal intercourse — as an unsafe sexual act, there will be a systematic underestimate of the act. A Wilcoxon ranks test reveals that, at least in this data set, this is not the case ($z = 0.02$, $p. = 0.98$).

Also, split-half reliability estimates of condom use show no significant differences between the samples (for insertive anal intercourse, $\chi^2 = 1.36$, $df = 2$, $p = 0.51$ and for receptive, $\chi^2 = 0.15$, $df = 2$, $p = 0.93$). Finally, a two-sample t test on the reliability of the estimates of number of sexual partners in the preceding year also yielded no significant differences (t-statistic $= 0.311$, $p = 0.76$). As a result of successful test-retest, consistency and split-half tests, we can be confident that the estimates provided by respondents are reliable.

Attrition

Attrition measures the loss of respondents from a longitudinal study as a result of both involuntary and voluntary factors. Involuntary departure from an ongoing study may occur because of illness or death, something which may be considered likely in a study which deliberately includes some respondents with a life threatening illness. Voluntary departure may occur for many reasons: subjects may weary of the annual interview procedure; some may find it too time consuming; circumstances may change which do not allow participation; some may move and simply forget to inform the project; still others may make a deliberate decision to leave the study because they disagree with methods or aims; and others may leave because they do not feel they are of sufficient interest to the study.

Attrition is considered important in longitudinal studies since a bias in key characteristics of those leaving the study may indicate that the general representativeness of the cohort is compromised. However, it may be that the overall representativeness of the cohort is questionable to start with, or at least not easily assessed. This consideration may well be much more important than the attrition characteristics as SIGMA probably suffers from bias in its representativeness for reasons we and others have rehearsed elsewhere.

All Sites

Tables 7.7 and 7.8 summarise the overall rates of attrition in the cohort. At the first phase 930 men were recruited to the cohort, 310 in London, 215 in Cardiff

Table 7.7. Summary of Interview Numbers

	Wave 1	Wave 2	Wave 3	Wave 4
Number interviewed	930			
Number reinterviewed as a percentage of wave 1		703 75.6	363 39.0	344 37.0
Deaths notified		1	11	6
Number of new recruits		52	11	78

Table 7.8. Recontacting Response by Site

	Wave 1	Wave 2	Wave 3	Wave 4
Cardiff % of wave 1	215	141 65.6	107 49.8	74 34.4
London % of wave 1	310	263 84.8	232 74.8	196 63.2
Newcastle and Teesside % of wave 1	138	104 75.4	— —	24 17.4
Norwich, Yorks and Portsmouth % of wave 1	132	108 81.8	— —	28 21.2
Birmingham, Bristol and Liverpool % of wave 1	135	87 64.4	9 —	27 20.0
London and Cardiff % of wave 1	525	404 76.9	339 64.6	270 51.4
Overall % of wave 1	930	703 75.6	363 39.0	344 37.5

and the remaining 405 elsewhere. In the second phase all were recontacted and 703 (75.6%) were reinterviewed. At the third phase only cohort respondents in Cardiff and London sites were recontacted and the overall response thus fell to 363 (39.0%). At the fourth phase all site respondents were recontacted and the overall response fell slightly to 349 (37.5%). Clearly the most significant factor affecting these numbers was the decision not to try to contact respondents outside London and Cardiff in the third phase of interviewing. If we break the figures down into their site components (Table 7.8), a much more impressive picture emerges. The response rates for London in each phase are 84.8%, 74.8% and 63.2%, and for Cardiff, 65.6%, 49.8% and 34.4%.

Taken together, the response rates for London and Cardiff, the only sites where respondents were consistently contacted, are 76.9%, 64.6% and 51.4%. Outside these two sites the response to invitations in the second phase was generally high, 82% being achieved in the London sites. The Cardiff sites only achieved a 64% return in this phase. By the fourth phase at least twenty-four months from

Table 7.9. Effect of Attrition on Key Sexual Behaviour Data

	Wave 2 mean (median)	Wave 4 mean (median)
Age		
Responders	32.9 (30)	34.9 (31)
Non-responders	29.4 (26)	30.4 (27)
	<.0001	<.0001
Numbers of partners		
Lifetime: Responders	300 (40)	360 (59)
Non-responders	212 (27)	231 (30)
	ns	ns
Lifetime PSP: Responders	84 (8)	85 (10)
Non-responders	63 (5)	75 (6)
	ns	ns
Last year: Responders	11 (4)	13 (5)
Non-responders	10 (4)	10 (4)
	ns	ns
Last year PSP: Responders	2.2 (1)	2.1 (1)
Non-responders	2.8 (1)	2.5 (1)
	ns	ns
Age of first homosexual sex		
Responders	15.6 (15)	16.1 (16)
Non-responders	15.3 (15)	15.1 (14)
	ns	ns
Gay relationship status		
	Percentages not responding	
Monogamous	30.6	70.2
Open relationship	21.4	59.2
Casuals only	22.8	61.4
	<.04	<.03

their last contact with the study for some of the subjects, a very low response is achieved in the sites outside Cardiff and London.

A comparison of the wave one characteristics of responders and non-responders to wave two reveals very few significant differences (Tables 7.9 and 7.10). Age is the most important variable distinguishing the two groups ($F_{1,927} = 14.87$, $p < .0001$): non-responders being younger (29.4 years) than responders (32.9 years). None of the sexual practice variables such as partner numbers, age at first homosexual experience, or engagement in any sexual activity, differentiates responders from non-responders except for gay relationship status where significantly more of those who were currently in monogamous relationships did not return for reinterview ($\chi^2 = 6.93$, df = 2, $p < .04$).

While characteristics such as sexual behaviour, marital status, behavioural bisexuality, homosexual disclosure and regret, ever considered discontinuing homosexual activities, how seriously you take safer sex and whether they had ever been HIV tested did not predict non-response, a few characteristics did.

Table 7.10. Variables on Which There Are Significant Differences in Attrition Rates

	Wave 2	Wave 4
	Proportions not responding	
Homosexual disclosure[1]		
None	32.1	67.9
Few	26.5	68.0
Half	23.7	71.2
Most	21.6	58.0
All	28.4	62.9
	ns	<.04
Perceived HIV status		
Tested positive	18.9	75.7
Thought positive	13.2	44.7
Tested negative but thought positive	25.0	33.3
Thought negative	22.9	62.4
Tested and thought negative	24.7	62.8
Don't know	51.1	83.0
	<.001	<.001
Highest educational qualification		
None	32.9	75.0
O level	31.2	71.7
A level	27.0	67.2
Hnd, etc.	29.7	68.5
Degree	14.9	53.8
Higher degree	10.5	37.1
	<.001	<.001
Behavioural bisexuality		
No	23.7	61.2
Yes	29.4	76.1
	ns	<.01

Note: [1] What proportion of your family and friends know you are gay/bisexual?

Responders are also more likely to have fewer educational qualifications ($\chi^2 = 31.78$, df = 5, p <. 0001): 32.9% of those with no qualifications not responding compared with just 10.5% of those with higher degrees. Of the HIV/AIDS variables analysed there is no significant difference between those who had previously had an HIV antibody test and those who had not, but perceived HIV status was significantly different ($\chi^2 = 21.93$, df = 5, p <. 0001). More than half of those who had no idea of their HIV status did not return compared with under a quarter in the other categories.

In a comparison of responders and non-responders in wave four, a similar pattern emerges. The remaining members of the cohort are those who were older in wave one (34.9 compared to 30.4) and they are better educated. Those who had disclosed their homosexuality to few of their friends, family and workmates were less likely to be still in the wave four cohort. Behavioural bisexuals (those with male and female partners in the preceding year) were less likely to respond to wave four, 76% of those in the original cohort failing to return by wave four compared to 61% of non-bisexuals ($\chi^2 = 8.56$, df = 1, p <. 01). Those in monogamous gay relationships were also least likely to stay with the study. With perceived HIV status, tested positives join don't knows as non-responders. On all key sexual behaviour variables there are no differences.

Attrition: Discussion

Overall, on most of the key variables there are no differences of particular note. Non-responders are least likely to disclose their homosexuality to others, which is as one might expect. They also tend to be younger, reflecting perhaps the greater mobility of this group who subsequently became more difficult to trace. Between waves three and four non-responders were more likely to be bisexual in feeling and actions; perhaps they came to see their sexual lifestyles as less important to a study of gay men (they may have stopped having sex with men).

The large differences in response rate geographically may be explained by different recall techniques and interviewer problems in the Cardiff site. It is unfair to look at the waves three and four response for all sites together since outside London and Cardiff the period between interview and recall was very long in waves two to four.

The non-response rate between waves is most pronounced between waves one and two for London and Cardiff and for all sites. Another large drop occurred between waves three and four. Some of this can be explained by subjects becoming bored or disillusioned with the study and by our own funding uncertainties at the third interview which meant we could not definitely tell subjects that a fourth interview would be required.

8 HIV Testing and Seroprevalence

As the preceding chapters have discussed, in the 1980s HIV had an immense impact on the lives of many gay men. During the last ten years discussions of safer sex, condom use and sexual negotiation have become part of the common currency of gay lifestyles. Similarly the issue of testing for HIV antibodies has been widely discussed, even though it has remained controversial ever since the antibody test became available in 1985. (The term 'HIV antibody' is used to indicate that the most common test, ELISA, looks for the body's antibodies to HIV, not for HIV itself. However, using the term 'HIV antibody test' is cumbersome, and for the rest of this chapter we will use the term 'HIV test'.)

For any individual, the decision to take an HIV test is fraught with difficulty and anxiety. Over the years the advantages and disadvantages have been well rehearsed in the gay press, though no consensus has emerged as yet. Two main reasons are advanced in favour of testing: that it helps to sustain safer sex; and, in the case of an HIV positive diagnosis, that it enables early medical intervention which may delay the progression to AIDS.

No study has produced incontrovertible evidence that being tested or knowing one's HIV status causes any long-term changes in sexual behaviour. However, two arguments are employed in support of this view: first, taking the test in itself indicates a degree of concern about HIV and the process of going to a clinic will involve counselling, and even if the man eventually declines the test, the process in itself may make him reflect on, and consequently alter, his sexual behaviour. Second, there is a presumption that knowing one's HIV status will reinforce safer sex behaviour. If a man tests negative, it is suggested he will redouble his efforts to remain negative by having only safer sex. If he tests positive, he may also redouble efforts not to infect others. Contrary arguments can, of course, be made. Someone testing positive may, for example, decide he doesn't care about infecting others, while a negative result after unsafe sexual behaviour may reinforce that behaviour.

Evidence from SIGMA suggests that whether or not a man engages in anal intercourse is unrelated to whether or not he's been tested. However, men who have tested positive are more likely to use condoms than men who don't know their serostatus or those who have tested negative.

The possibility of early medical intervention in men found to be positive is a reason for testing given by many members of the medical profession. Giving

Figure 8.1. Perceived Advantages and Disadvantages of HIV Antibody Testing

Advantages	Disadvantages
Peace of mind Early medical intervention Can plan changes in lifestyle Reinforces safer sex	Difficulty of coping with positive result Fear of stigma/rejection and discrimination Problems getting insurance Encourages complacency regarding safer sex

AZT for asymptomatic HIV, it is argued, may slow progression to symptomatic states (the 'Concorde' trial, which is investigating this hypothesis, reports after we go to press). Furthermore, some prophylactic treatments against opportunistic infections may be of help, such as Septrin or nebulised pentamidine against the common respiratory infection PCP. However, trials testing the effectiveness of anti-virals in asymptomatic people with HIV have still to be concluded, and the use of prophylaxis early in the disease against opportunistic infections is still to be assessed. Given the relative uncertainty of the benefits of early intervention, it is wholly understandable that some men take this as but one consideration when deciding whether to test for HIV or not.

The Individual Decision

The decision to take an HIV test is something all gay men have faced from time to time since one became available. It is never an easy decision particularly because it raises questions about how to cope with the result. Men in this study recognise that there are both advantages and disadvantages in having a test. These reasons were nearly always qualified by the likely outcome. Figure 8.1 summarises the main advantages and disadvantages given by men. The majority saw clear advantages in knowing a positive result. Important practical plans could be made for the future, including seeking early medical interventions and making changes to lifestyles. However, the majority also saw clear disadvantages about knowing a positive result. In particular, more than half were concerned that they would not be able to cope and that the anxiety would have a deleterious effect on their health.

Not surprisingly, the prospect of receiving a negative result was less problematic. Some claimed it would affirm their current safer sex lifestyles, but a smaller number thought it could undermine their own commitment to safer sex by making them complacent. Very few mentioned the procedure of being tested and the uncertainty and anxiety of awaiting a result as a disadvantage, but a few were worried that a test result could be misused.

Of those who had tested most said they had done so for peace of mind,

Figure 8.2. Perceived HIV Status

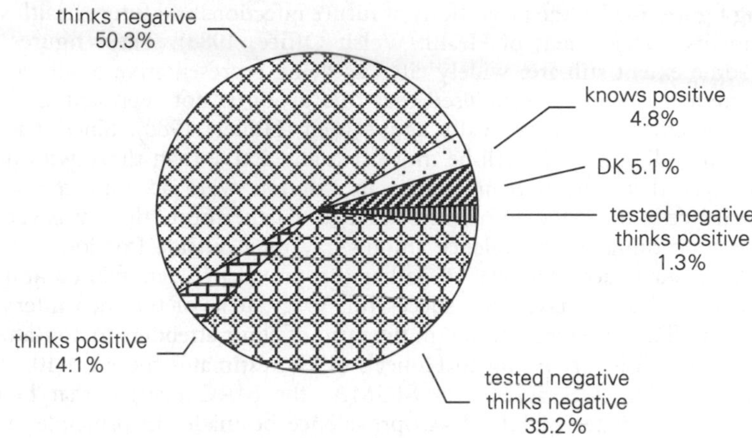

especially if they were worried about past unsafe behaviour. Less than a tenth mentioned courtship as a reason, although this is reputedly an important consideration in parts of the USA. Very few were tested because they felt unwell. For those who had decided not to be tested, nearly half said this was because they did not consider that they were at risk and would almost certainly test negative. A further fifth had decided not to get a test because they were afraid of the repercussions of a positive test result. About a tenth had decided not to test because of perceived anxiety while awaiting the result. Men who had most partners, especially casuals, were more likely to have been tested, as were men who thought themselves to be positive and those who engaged in anal intercourse. All these factors add to the view that clinic-based estimates of HIV seroprevalence among gay men are likely to be gross overestimates.

Just over half the men in this study have been tested at least once, and about a quarter have been tested more than once. Most had the test at a GUM or STD clinic rather than by a GP. The proportion who have taken a test in the year before each interview has not changed much over the period of study.

At each interview we ask what people think their status is irrespective of whether they have taken a test or not. As Figure 8.2 illustrates, the majority (over 85%) consistently believe that they are HIV antibody negative. A smaller number (about 5%) know they are positive, and a similar number think they are positive but have not had a positive result. The most common reason these men give for believing they are positive is past or current unsafe sex, followed by current poor health.

The Seroprevalence Study

In the UK studies of HIV seroprevalence among gay men have invariably been based on men who attend STD clinics (Carne *et al.*, 1987; Department of Health/Welsh Office, 1988; Evans *et al.*, 1989). In 1987, as the project was starting, reports from GUM clinics in London suggested that about a quarter of all gay men being (voluntarily) tested for antibodies to HIV were positive (Carne *et al.*, 1987). Such alarming figures fuelled the projections of future infections and future health service requirements (Department of Health/Welsh Office, 1988). These figures were, and to some extent still are, widely cited as being representative of all gay men, even though it is widely recognised that this group is not representative of the whole population of homosexually active men (Hillier, 1988). Since it is likely that men attending a clinic will be more sexually active than those who do not, it is unlikely that figures from clinics in London were accurate measures of seroprevalence in the gay communities at large. Furthermore, there was very little evidence concerning seroprevalence among gay men outside London.

One of our major aims was to gather seroprevalence data from a non-clinic cohort and in this we have been successful. Only 40% of the men interviewed were regular clinic attenders, although the ratio of clinic attenders to non-attenders in the population is, according to Hillier's (1988) estimates, nearer 1:10.

When funding was agreed for SIGMA, the MRC insisted that blood be collected and estimates of HIV-1 seroprevalence be made. In principle, a study recruiting from non-clinic sources should give a more accurate picture of seroprevalence in the gay communities generally and would provide estimates both for London and for South Wales (the original MRC funded sites). This requirement required the research team to become trained HIV counsellors and phlebotomists. This training, over several days, was given at King's College Hospital in South London. The general reaction from the research team was favourable, though one refused to take blood. This requirement also made the research difficult to insure and caused some local problems with ethical committees and university/polytechnic regulations regarding storage of needles and sharps. A sample of blood from all research members taking blood was also stored in case of later needle-stick injury.

At an early stage it was decided that if a respondent wanted their HIV test result, they should be given it, but that otherwise they would not be informed of their result. The decision to make the result available was taken on the grounds that this was something we could offer respondents, but should not be taken to indicate that the project had a pro-testing stance. This was particularly important in Cardiff where the local GUM clinic historically had a poor reputation in the gay communities. Pre-test counselling (before blood was taken) generally proceeded clarifying what the result could and could not tell, discussing the advantages and disadvantages of getting a result and taking the respondent through how they would react if the test came back positive. Respondents were, where appropriate, referred to specialist agencies.

No-one was pressurised into giving blood, but at each wave about two-thirds did so. A system was put in place in both sites for giving respondents results, if they specifically requested the information, and then only after counselling about the implications. In London they were referred to Dr T.J. McManus, a principal investigator and consultant in genitourinary medicine at King's College Hospital (south-east London), and in Cardiff Professor Coxon gave results. Approximately 40–70% of respondents asked for their HIV test result, depending on wave number and geographical location. The figure for Cardiff was somewhat higher than London, partly because some men used the project as an alternative testing site.

The testing was carried out at the PHLS Laboratory in Dulwich Hospital, south London, to which samples were delivered by post. Bloods were screened initially by a competitive enzyme immunoassay (ELISA) for HIV antibodies (Wellcozyme, Wellcome), and positively reacting sera were confirmed by an indirect ELISA (Anti-HIV, second generation, Abbott). If necessary, further confirmatory tests were carried out at another HIV reference centre. Before a respondent gave a sample of blood, an informed consent form had to be signed (Coxon *et al.*, 1992). We also asked some respondents for a small saliva sample which was tested at the same time for HIV antibodies as part of a study to assess the effectiveness of saliva testing (this is discussed in more detail below). At the first three waves testing was carried out only in London and Cardiff. In the fourth wave this was extended to all sites. This necessitated much additional travelling for the researchers since an extra journey had to be made to give HIV results to men requesting them from sites all over the country.

Confidentiality was of prime importance with the HIV results. SIGMA had a clear policy on storage of results and access to them. Consequently, bloods were marked only with the respondent number, a unique series of a two-letter site code and a four-digit number. This number could only be linked to a person's name and address in one file on a secure PC, password protected. No other data were linked to the blood data. The results were initially only accessible to the principal investigators, and analysis only proceeded once the identifiers had been stripped from the data files. In the third and fourth wave access was given to the senior researchers, a practical move following the departure of two of the principal investigators to other universities. These procedures were explained to respondents and our guarantees of confidentiality were generally approved and accepted, al though a few men did refuse a blood sample on these grounds.

Seroprevalence of HIV-1

Here we describe the basic findings of the seroprevalence study: overall seroprevalence of HIV and differences between London and Cardiff. We also compare prevalence among clinic and non-clinic attenders and discuss some of the characteristics of those testing HIV positive.

All the men interviewed in London and South Wales (in wave one n = 525) were asked to give a sample of blood for testing for HIV. At each stage about two-thirds did so. Apart from the fact that those agreeing were slightly younger than men who refused, there were no other statistically significant differences between respondents who agreed to be bled and those who did not. For example, men providing us with a sample of blood were neither more nor less likely to have taken the test previously, nor more likely to be clinic attenders.

Nine per cent of the men interviewed in London tested positive at the first interview (1987) compared to $3\frac{1}{2}$ % in South Wales, giving an overall rate of 7%. Adjusting this for men who had past positive results but who SIGMA did not test and for those who were tested negative elsewhere during the course of interviewing, the figures rise to 14% within London and $4\frac{1}{2}$ % in Cardiff (Hunt *et al.*, 1990).

Just under a third of the men either described themselves as regular GUM clinic attenders or had attended a GUM clinic in the year preceding interview.

Table 8.1. Numbers of Partners and PSPs of Seronegatives and Seropositives

	Negatives				Positives			
	Mean	Median	Upper quartile	Lower quartile	Mean	Median	Upper quartile	Lower quartile
Whole life								
Partners	452.7	50	15	250	528.7	200	40	800
PSPS	99.4	10	2	30	198.0	50	6	480
Last five years								
Partners	64.2	20	7	50	144.4	40	17	150
PSPS	10.2	3	1	9	46.3	17	4	40
Last year								
Partners	13.8	6	2	14	24.6	6	3	22
PSPS	2.5	1	0	2	5.9	1	0	7
Last month								
Partners	2.1	1	1	3	3.1	1	0	4
PSPS	0.5	0	0	1	1.0	0	0	1

These clinic attenders reported higher numbers of partners and PSPS, and were more likely to test HIV antibody positive (overall 16% against 4%). Thus figures based solely on information from GUM clinics will overstate the proportion of gay men who have HIV. This result is partly explained by the fact that those who are tested at clinics tend to be more sexually active and to think of themselves at risk. It is also the case that having symptoms of HIV-related illness is sometimes the reason men go to a clinic to be tested.

The rate of seropositivity among men who had previously been tested was higher than for those not previously tested (13.8% against 5.8%). Taken together, these figures suggest that the rate of HIV infection among gay and bisexual men in the UK is substantially lower than that suggested by clinic studies.

Individual characteristics such as age, disclosure of homosexuality or marital status do not distinguish those who tested positive from those who tested negative. Clinicians who use such factors to judge the probability of a positive result or insurance or mortgage companies who make decisions on these bases are misguided. As Table 8.1 demonstrates, men who reported higher numbers of PSPs were most likely to test positive, reporting on average more than twice the number of PSPs of those testing negative. Although men testing positive also tended to have more partners than those testing negative, there was not a significant difference. All the men who tested positive had engaged in anal intercourse previously, and no-one who had not done so tested positive.

As Table 8.2 illustrates, a past history of syphilis was also closely linked to a positive result: 37% of men who tested positive had had syphilis in the past compared to 12% of those testing negative. Similarly the positive group reported three times as many occurrences of infection episodes as those testing negative. Of course, this is most likely because men with a history of syphilis report higher numbers of PSPs. This association does mean that syphilis might be a useful marker of men having anal intercourse. It is also the case that men with HIV are very likely to have hepatitis B, CMV or herpes, though in the case of herpes at

Table 8.2. Characteristics of Those Testing Negative and Positive to HIV Antibody

	London Cohort		
	Tested positive N = 19	Tested negative N = 187	Significance
Age (median)	32	29	NS
Age (mean)	31.2	33.0	
Regular partners	13 (68.4%)	92 (49.2%)	NS
Disclosure	76.%	84.%	NS
Previous history of syphilis	7 (36.8%)	22 (12.2%)	<0.01
Mean number of episodes of syphilis	0.37	0.12	<0.05
Herpes	5 (26.3%)	17 (9.1%)	<0.05

least, this may simply reflect the fact that it is a common HIV-related opportunistic infection. Although many other STDs were reported, none was linked to HIV status.

HIV-1 Seroconversions

A further aim was to estimate seroconversion rates over the period of study. Eleven men who tested negative for HIV antibodies in wave one became positive during the course of the study (Hunt *et al.*, 1992). A detailed consideration of the interview data allows us to make fair estimates of dates of seroconversion and to examine sexual practices and relationships immediately prior to this. All had engaged in unprotected anal intercourse, either receptive or insertive or both. While this is not conclusive proof that this is how they were infected, since all will have performed other sexual practices, it is instructive that no-one who always used condoms for anal intercourse, or who had not engaged, seroconverted. Furthermore, eight of the men almost certainly became infected by fucking with a regular partner, four of whom were known to be positive at the time.

There were no time trends observable in the small numbers, and therefore we cannot say whether the rate of seroconversions has increased or decreased.

Saliva Testing for HIV-1

Measurements of the prevalence of HIV-1, an essential element in the epidemiological study of the spread of HIV-1, are reliably made from samples of blood. In the setting of the clinic or hospital environment this presents few problems, but many epidemiological studies of marginalised groups, such as male and female sex workers or injecting drug users, do not have access to phlebotomy services as much fieldwork is carried out outside a clinic setting. Consequently, the application of a non-invasive method for HIV testing is desirable. Equally importantly, some people find the giving of blood traumatic and may refuse to cooperate in the study. With these points in mind saliva tests for anti-HIV-1 antibodies have been developed (Parry, 1986; Parry *et al.*, 1987) and proven in clinical trials to be effective (Johnson *et al.*, 1988). To validate fully the saliva test in the non-clinic

Table 8.3. HIV-1 Antibody Tests on Saliva/Blood Pairs of Samples

	Wave 1	Wave 2	All tests	Percentage
Blood and saliva negative	273	214	487	94.60
Blood and saliva positive	17	8	25	4.80
Saliva positive blood negative	0	0	0	0.00
Saliva negative blood positive	1	0	1	0.20
Equivocal*	2	0	2	0.04
Total tested	293	222	515	100.00
Insufficient sample	11	8	19	
Total collected	304	230	534	

Note: * Two tests were equivocal, that is, the saliva result for two positive bloods could not exclude a positive result.

environment, it needs to be shown that saliva samples can be collected by non-medical personnel and that the saliva samples collected correspond with the blood tests.

Taking advantage of the blood study, we ran a study to test the reliability of a saliva test in a field research setting (Hunt *et al.*, 1993). Although HIV is not thought to be carried in saliva, antibodies can be detected in it. Everyone bled in waves one and two was asked for a sample of saliva, obtained by chewing on a piece of cotton which was then sealed and sent, with the respondent number attached, for testing at the PHLS (Colindale). Only those salivas for which we had a blood result were used in the analysis, although as a general screening measure some non-bleeders were asked to provide saliva. No-one was given an HIV antibody result from the saliva test.

As Table 8.3 illustrates, this study proved that it was possible to collect samples of saliva and get them to the testing station, and that the saliva test was both sensitive and specific. In other words, the saliva test did not fail to find positives (sensitivity); nor did it falsely label negative results positive (specificity).

9 Parameters of Sexual Behaviour

Well, tell it like it is, and how it could be,
How it was, and of course how it should be,
Let's talk about sex!
Salt and Pepa ('Let's talk about sex', 1991)

In this chapter we look at the broad outlines of individual sexual experience: first sexual experiences; the lifetime sexual repertoire; and current sexual behaviours including condom use and sexual behaviour with females. Finally, we look at overall numbers of sexual partners, and penetrative sexual partners, a matter of great concern to epidemiologists.

First Sexual Experiences

As we have seen in Chapter 2, gay liberation in the 1970s made coming out the central moral and political prescription for the movement. In the 1970s and 1980s a great deal of work was done by gay scholars and others on the process of 'coming out', the process whereby an individual realised the potential of his or her sexuality (see, for example, Cass, 1984; Troiden, 1988). Behind this research lie both descriptive and prescriptive agenda. On the one hand, it is an attempt to codify and explain an important — arguably the most important — facet of individual gay experience; and on the other, it seeks to provide a template for successful management of self. Coming out becomes more than a psychological process; it becomes a subculturally validated rite of passage.

There has been much debate over the role of sexual experience in the coming out process. At the heart of this debate is the problem of seduction. The Wolfenden Report (Home Office/Scottish Home Department, 1957) set great store by the need to protect young men from the attentions of older men and from their own inexperience. The idea that young men and boys can be seduced into a homosexual lifestyle has a long history (for review, see Plummer, 1975). Seeking to shed light on this problem, we asked respondents to describe in some detail their first homosexual and heterosexual experiences and in particular to say whether they were expected or 'hoped for'.

Figure 9.1 presents graphically the age at which they first suspected they were

Figure 9.1. Age Suspect Sexually Different (A); Label That Difference Gay (B); First Sex with a Man (C); and First Anal Intercourse (D)

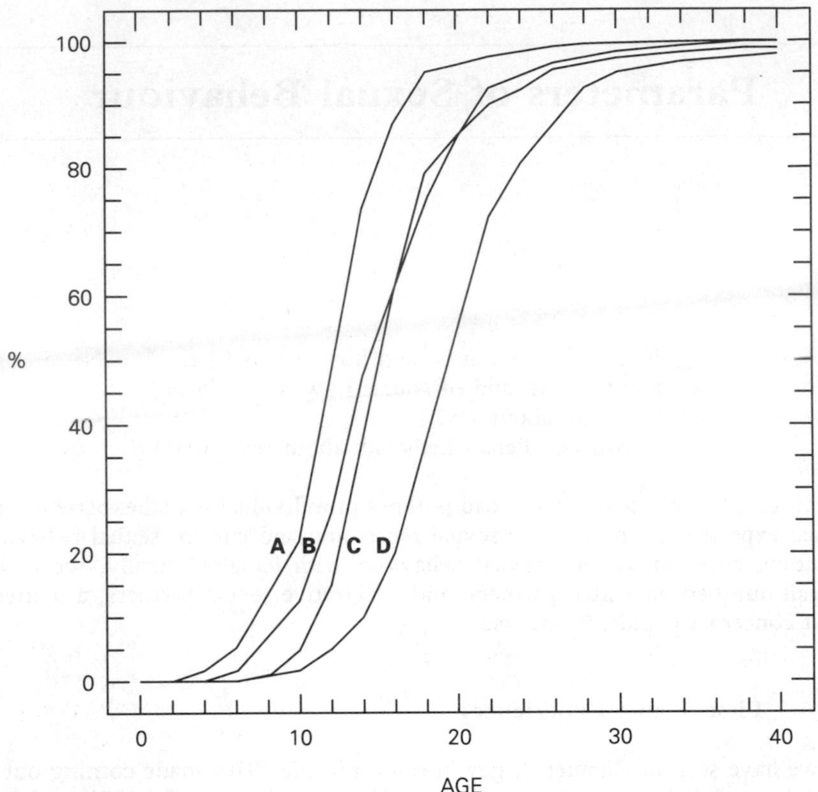

sexually different (A); labelled that difference homosexual or gay (B); had their first sexual experience with a man (C); and first experience of anal intercourse (D).

Nearly a quarter (22%) suspected they were sexually different before they were 10 years of age, and almost all (97%) did so before they were 20.
Some (10%) realised they were gay before they were 10 years of age, and the majority (86%) did so before they were 20.
Over a quarter (26%) engaged in homosexual sex before they suspected they were sexually different.
Very few (3%) had their first sexual experiences with another man before they were 10, but the vast majority (87%) did so before they were 20.
The majority (67%) engaged in homosexual sex only after they had labelled themselves as gay (or homosexual).

It therefore seems that for the majority of these men their first (homo)sexual experience confirmed or validated an existing sexual preference or identity. It is also apparent that during the teenage years most go through a period of realisation of sexual difference, a labelling process and at least the beginnings of coming out.

Almost none (<1%) had their first experience of anal intercourse before they were 10, but more than half (56%) did so before they were 20.
The average (mean) age at first homosexual experience was 15.7 years.
The average (mean) age of first experience of anal intercourse was 20.9 years.

These findings point to the fact that anal intercourse is not the staple feature of the male homosexual repertoire that common folklore would have us believe, a fact that we take up in some detail later in this chapter and again in Chapter 10.

The median age difference between partners, at first sex, was one year.
40% of first experiences are with men of the same age, and almost 60% with partners less than two years older or younger.
20% first had sex with a man who was 10 years or more older than themselves.
Most hoped for their first encounter; many actively sought it.
Less than 1% of these first sexual experiences were non-consensual.

As we have stressed, the Wolfenden Report (Home Office/Scottish Home Department, 1957) showed great concern over the ability of young men to resist both advances from older men and their own poor judgment. On these figures it appears that a fifth, at most, had their first experience with a much older man, but the evidence suggest that a much smaller proportion could be claimed to be the victims of older predatory 'homosexuals'. That is, although almost 90% of these men had their first homosexual experience before it was legal for them to do so, these data do not support the idea of homosexual 'recruitment' or seduction as the means by which individuals are introduced to homosexual sex and the gay subculture. Rather, they support the contention that sexual experiences follow the recognition of homosexual attraction and, to a slightly lesser extent, gay identity formation.

Lifetime Sexual Repertoire

Despite popular conflations of 'gay sex' with bizarre or unnatural sexual practices, among very many respondents there is a clear preference for a small number of fairly unremarkable sexual acts. However, the lifetime sexual repetoire of some of the men involves a wide diversity of sexual behaviours.

All respondents were asked to provide information about all the sexual activities that they had *ever* engaged in, with another man. The cumulative experience or repertoire, displayed in Table 9.1, gives some indication of the range of behaviours and the differential popularity of some of the acts. The pattern which emerges is of three core groups of activities: those that virtually all the men (95%+) have engaged in (the *common*); a group of acts the vast majority of the men (75–90%) have engaged in (the *fairly common*); and a final group of acts that less than half the men have ever engaged in, aptly named the uncommon.

Very nearly all had engaged in self-masturbation.

Table 9.1. Percentages Ever Engaging in Sex Acts, Percentages Doing So in Last Month and, for Those Doing So, the Mean Number of Times in Last Month

	Sex act	percentage ever	percentage per Month	Average (mean)
Common	**Masturbation**			
	Self	99½	90	17
	Passive	95	63	7
	Active	96	66	7
	Fellatio	*97	*68	
	Insertive	96	58	7
	Receptive	95	61	7
	Kissing	96	67	12
Fairly common	**Anal fingering**	90	42	3
	Body rubbing	84	52	4
	Anal intercourse	*92	*41	
	Receptive	85	28	3
	Insertive	85	29	3
	Massage	81	41	4
	Anilingus	81	31	3
	Inter-femoral	78	30	3
Uncommon	**Corporal Punishment**	41	10	2
	Lindinism	28	3	2
	Brachio-proctic	17	1	2
	Douching	7	1	2
	Coprophilia	3	0	0

Note: * These are the percentages engaging in *either* insertive *or* receptive or both.

The horror at nocturnal pollution and the spending of semen is a consistent feature of Christian and thus Western thought. During the nineteenth century and well into the twentieth, masturbation was regarded as a particularly pernicious vice. Krafft-Ebing (1925: *passim*), for example, sought to explain the emergence of the paraphilias as a result of masturbation. As a result, a wide range of truly frightening instruments were on general sale for parents to prevent children from masturbating. Though still something of a taboo topic, in recent years masturbation has begun to be regarded with much less horror, and some contemporary sex education programs come close to recommending it for both boys and girls.

Almost all (95%+) had masturbated, fellated and deep kissed another man.

The implication of anal intercourse in HIV transmission has naturally focused attention on other facets of the homosexual repertoire. The evidence that exists, however, suggests that masturbation and fellatio were always among the most common features of the homosexual repertoire (Westwood, 1960; Schofield, 1965a; Bell and Weinberg, 1978).

> Between 70% and 90% have engaged in inter-femoral intercourse, anilingus, body rubbing, massage, anal fingering and anal intercourse.
> Although less than half have engaged in any of the other acts, they too form part of the lifetime sexual repertoire of many men.

As we have seen, many of the early causal explanations of HIV infection focused on the unnatural or fast-lane activities of gay men. These included anal intercourse, but also acts such as fisting and water sports. Therefore, it is important to note the relative unpopularity of some of these sexual activities. Thus, while these activities may be more popular than they are among the exclusively heterosexual population (and this must remain supposition until data become available), they should not be considered a prerequisite, or even a common feature of homosexual experience. Of particular note is the fact that:

> anal intercourse is not universally practised, and a significant proportion of men have never engaged in this activity.

Current Sexual Behaviour

Lifetime repertoire may include acts which are staples of sexual activity as well as others that featured only once or twice. All respondents were asked to provide information about their sexual behaviour in the month preceding each interview. Table 9.1 displays these percentages. It is particularly noticeable that the general pattern of common, fairly common and uncommon acts recurs, though of course the percentages involved are smaller.

> The most common activity (90%) is self-masturbation.
> About two-thirds currently engaged in kissing, masturbation and fellatio.
> About a third engaged in body rubbing, massage, fingering and anal intercourse, and about a quarter in anilingus and inter-crural intercourse.
> No more than one in ten had engaged in most of the other acts.

Of particular note is the fact that:

> anal intercourse is by no means the most common current sexual activity.

As we shall see, these figures are affected by a range of factors, but overall the pattern remains clear.

All respondents who had engaged in each act were also asked to recall how often they had done so in the month preceding interview. Again the same broad pattern appears; Table 9.1 also displays the mean number of times respondents had engaged in each act in the last month.

> Men who had sex by themselves did so, on average, fifteen to eighteen times a month.

While the only common solitary sexual activity was masturbation, a wide range of accompaniments was used, including sexually explicit materials, such as videos and magazines, and a variety of lubricants and toys.

> Men who had sex with another man did so, on average, eight to ten times a month.

As we shall see below, this overall figure is heavily influenced by the type of sexual relationship the men were involved in.

> Sex with other men is most likely to involve masturbation, fellatio and deep kissing.

For a vast majority of the men all these sexual activities occur in more or less all their sexual sessions. Moreover, since deep kissing alone was not considered sufficient to classify that interaction as sexual, it is commonly reported to have occurred on more occasions than there were sex sessions.

> Acts such as anal intercourse, fingering, massage, body rubbing, anilingus or inter-femoral intercourse appear in less than half of sexual sessions.

Even among men who engage in any of the other sexual activities, none do so as frequently, with all these activities appearing in fewer than half of men's sexual sessions.
It is important to note that:

> anal intercourse is not a particularly frequent part of the sexual repertoire, even among men who currently engage in the activity.

Patterns of Engagement in Anal Intercourse

In the previous section we reported that a significant proportion of gay men have never engaged in anal intercourse; that anal intercourse is by no means the most common current sexual activity; and, finally, that anal intercourse is not a particularly frequent part of the sexual repertoire, even among men who currently engage in it.

However, for two disparate but very important reasons, anal intercourse is the sexual activity that is of central importance to this book. First, anal intercourse has repeatedly been proven the most efficient means of sexual transmission of HIV, at least among men (Detels *et al.*, 1983; Goedert *et al.*, 1984, 1985; Melbye *et al.*, 1984; Marmor *et al.*, 1984; Groopman *et al.*, 1985; Nicholson *et al.*, 1985; Jeffries *et al.*, 1985; Mayer *et al.*, 1986; Schechter *et al.*, 1986; Stevens *et al.*, 1986; Chmiel *et al.*, 1987; Darrow *et al.*, 1987; Kingsley *et al.*, 1987; Moss *et al.*, 1987; van Griensven *et al.*, 1987; Winkelstein *et al.*, 1987; Coates *et al.*, 1988; McCusker *et al.*, 1988; Osmond *et al.*, 1988; Hunt *et al.*, 1991). Second, anal intercourse is commonly presumed to have a significance beyond the purely physical (Prieur, 1990; Hickson *et al.*, 1992), a subject we will return to in depth in Chapter 10.

Table 9.2. Insertive and Receptive Anal Intercourse with Regular and Casual Partnors in the Last Year (upper percentages are row-wise, lower are column-wise)

N = 330	Insertive with regular only (n = 123)	Insertive with both regular and casual (n = 96)	Insertive with casual only (n = 55)	Insertive with neither (n = 56)
Receptive with regular only (n = 140)	81 57.9% 65.9%	23 16.4% 24.0%	7 5.0% 12.7%	29 20.7% 51.8%
Receptive with both regular and casual (n = 72)	10 13.9% 8.1%	43 59.7% 44.8%	7 9.7% 12.7%	12 16.7% 21.4%
Receptive with casual only (n = 45)	1 2.2% 0.8%	8 17.7% 8.3%	21 46.7% 38.2%	15 33.4% 26.8%
Receptive with neither (n = 73)	31 42.5% 25.2%	22 30.1% 22.9%	20 27.4% 36.4%	—

For both these reasons, and because the monthly figures cited above underestimate the rates in any given year, the patterns of engagement in anal intercourse of the 468 men who participated in wave four (1991–92) are examined below. Table 9.2 shows the sixteen possible combinations of being insertive and receptive with regular and casual partners (for definitions of regular and casual partners see Chapter 11). In Table 9.2 of which the bottom right-hand cell is empty, but would contain the 138 men who had not fucked, we can see that in any given year more than two-thirds (70.5%) of gay men fuck. Overall, in the year before the wave four interview 70.5% (n = 330) of men had engaged in anal intercourse. Of these 58.5% (n = 274) had done so with a regular partner and 40.4% (n = 189) had done so with a casual partner.

Fucking is more common with regular partners than with casuals.

Of the men who had fucked 42.7% (n = 141) had done so only with regular partners, compared to 16.7% (n = 56) who had done so only with casuals, and 40.3% (n = 133) with both regulars and casuals.

Most men who fuck do so both ways.

Engaging in anal intercourse both receptively and insertively is more common than either one or the other: 60.9% (n = 201) had done both, 22.1% (n = 73) had been insertive only, and 17.0% (n = 56) had been receptive only. The most common patterns were to be both insertive and receptive with regular partners only (24.5%; n = 81), followed by 13.0% (n = 43) who do so both ways with both partner types.

Role specificity (only fucking one way) is more common than reciprocity (fucking both ways) among those who had only casual partners.

Table 9.3. The Percentage Engaging in Each Sexual Act in the Last Month by Relationship Status

Sexual act	Monogamous	Relationship Status Open	No regular	Significance
Masturbation				
Self	87	89	92	NS
Passive	69	75	50	<.001
Active	72	79	52	<.001
Fellatio				
Insertive	68	72	42	<.001
Receptive	76	77	39	<.001
Body rubbing				
Passive	48	45	27	<.001
Active	48	50	31	<.001
Anal intercourse				
Receptive	34	38	16	<.001
Insertive	38	39	16	<.001

Nearly two-thirds (62.5%) of those with only casual partners were role-specific compared to 42.6% of those with only regular partners. This could be because fucking with casuals is less common, and sex is likely to occur only once, so the opportunity for reciprocity is diminished, but see the discussion of power in anal intercourse in Chapter 10.

Factors Affecting Current Sexual Behaviour

Our pilot work (Coxon, 1986) and the work of others (Bell and Weinberg, 1978; Connell *et al.*, 1989) had suggested two factors that can be considered key determinants of sexual behaviour: how old someone is, whether they have a steady, or regular partner. Hence we will examine the incidence and frequency of specific sexual behaviours within different types of sexual relationship and age groups.

To simplify the rest of this chapter, we will concentrate on masturbation, fellatio, body rubbing, anal intercourse, anilingus, and inter-crural intercourse, the six most common acts which are implicated in many safer sex messages.

Effects of Relationship Status

The main predictor of current engagement in any sexual act is relationship status. As Tables 9.3 and 9.4 demonstrate, the key difference is between those men who have a regular sexual partner and these who do not.

Men in regular relationships are:

> more likely to engage in each of the sex acts. For example, in the preceding month: 39% of men in regular relationships fucked a man compared to 16% of men who had no regular sexual partner; 77% of men in regular relationships sucked a man compared to 39% of those who had no regular sexual partner.

Table 9.4. The Mean Monthly Frequency of Engagement in Each Sexual Act by Relationship Status (for those who engaged in the act)

Sexual act	Monogamous	Relationship Status Open	No regular	Significance
Masturbation				
Self	14	18	19	<.001
Passive	9	8	5	<.001
Active	9	8	5	<.001
Fellatio				
Insertive	8	7	4	<.001
Receptive	8	7	4	<.001
Body rub				
Passive	6	5	4	<.01
Active	5	5	4	<.01
Anal intercourse				
Receptive	4	3	2	<.001
Insertive	3	3	2	<.01

and, when they do so, they do so more frequently than men without regular partner. For example, in the preceding month: men in regular relationships who were fucked did so twice as often (four times) as men who did so, but had no regular partner; men in regular relationships who wanked a man did so twice as often (nine times) as men who did so, but had no regular sexual partner.

Men in monogamous relationships are:

slightly less likely to engage in each of the sex acts. For example, in the preceding month: 69% of men in monogamous relationships wanked another man compared to 75% of men in open regular relationships;

but when they do engage in any activity,

they do so slightly more frequently than men in open relationships. For example, in the preceding month: men in monogamous relationships who were sucked by another man did so eight times compared to seven times for men who had an open relationship.

Predictably, self-masturbation reverses these patterns. Men in regular (especially monogamous) relationships masturbate themselves considerably less than the others.

Effects of Age Group on Sexual Behaviour

Age group is far less important than relationship status as a predictor of engagement in any sexual act. However, age does have some effect on the types and quantity of sexual acts engaged in, though not a significant effect on risk taking behaviour, as is commonly presumed (see Davies *et al.*, 1992, for description of

Table 9.5. The Percentage Engaging in Each Sexual Act in the Last Month by Age Group

Sexual act	Under 21	Age Group 21–30	31–40	40+	Significance
Masturbation					
Self	86	92	94	81	<.0001
Passive	68	66	60	57	NS
Active	66	68	64	63	NS
Fellatio					
Insertive	64	64	54	46	<.001
Receptive	63	66	57	53	NS
Body rub					
Passive	41	42	37	30	NS
Active	41	46	40	35	NS
Anal intercourse					
Receptive	36	30	24	23	NS
Insertive	34	29	28	293	NS

Table 9.6. *The Mean Monthly Frequency Engagement in Each Sexual Act of by Age Group (for those who engaged in the act)*

Sexual act	Under 21	Age Group 21–30	31–40	40+	Significance
Masturbation					
Self	15	19	19	14	<.001
Passive	8	7	8	5	<.01
Active	8	8	8	6	NS
Fellatio					
Insertive	8	7	7	5	NS
Receptive	8	7	7	5	NS
Body rub					
Passive	6	5	4	3	NS
Active	4	4	3	3	NS
Anal intercourse					
Receptive	4	3	3	4	NS
Insertive	4	3	3	3	NS

the sexual behaviour of under-21-year-olds). As Tables 9.5 and 9.6 demonstrate, the key difference is between the men under 30 years of age and those older than that.

> Over 40s are the least sexually active. They are least likely to engage in any given act. For example, in the preceding month: 46% of over 40s were sucked by a man compared to between 54% and 64% of all the other age groups; and, when they do engage in any given act, they do so least often. For example, in the preceding month: over 40s who wanked another man did so six times compared to an average of eight times for the other age groups.
>
> Under 21s are most sexually active; they are most likely to engage in any given act. For example, in the preceding month: 34% of under 21s fucked

> another man compared to between 28% and 29% of the other age groups; and, when they do engage in any given act, they do so most often. For example, in the preceding month: under 21s who were sucked by another man did so eight times compared to an average of between five and seven times for the other age groups.
>
> For the most common acts (masturbation, fellatio, body rubbing, anal intercourse) there is an age gradient. Under 21s are more active than the 21–30s, who are more active than the over 30s, who are more active than the over 40s.

For the less common activities (not displayed in tabular form) the 21–30s are most likely to engage and have the highest frequencies, followed by the under 21s. This suggests that some of the less common acts might be learnt, or at least practised, later in the sexual career.

Geographical Location

Where men live (within or outside London) had no significant effect on which sexual activities men engaged in, or the number of times they did so.

Comment

For most men, most of the time sexual behaviour consists predominantly of masturbation, fellatio and body rubbing. Although anal intercourse is not universally practised, it still forms part of the sexual repertoire of a large proportion of homosexually active men. Beyond these, there is a wide range of sexual activities that figure prominently in the repertoires of a few men, infrequently in those of many others, but not at all in the repertoire of the majority of gay men.

Although the statistics summarise a wide range of frequencies, the figures confirm Kinsey *et al.*'s (1948: 632) assertion that 'even when the calculations are confined to those males who are having actual experience, the average frequencies are never high.' Clearly, these data lend no support to the idea that the norm for homosexually active men is to be hypersexually active.

Of the two factors presumed to influence the incidence and the frequency of engagement in sexual activity, by far the strongest and most consistent is type of sexual relationship. While there are differences in mean frequencies between those in a monogamous relationship and those who have an open relationship, the key difference is between those who have a regular sexual relationship and those who do not. The latter engage far less often in all sexual acts, presumably because they have less easy, and/or less productive access to sexual outlets.

Variation in the incidence and frequency data by relationship type suggests that much sexual activity is sexual partner (or at least partnership type) specific. This supports the idea that sexual activity can only be understood by taking account, not only of both those individuals involved but of the nature of their interaction and the social and psychic context of the sexual encounter (Davies and Weatherburn, 1991).

Table 9.7. Condom Use for Insertive Anal Intercourse (for those who engaged in anal intercourse in the last month)

	Total n	Always	Never (percentages)	Sometimes
All	270	38.9	49.6	11.5
Partner type[1]				
Regular	210	33.8	57.6	8.6
Casual	39	69.2	20.5	10.3
Relationship type				
Monogamous	93	28.0	59.1	12.9
Open	177	44.6	44.6	10.7
Age group				
<21	38	42.1	44.7	13.2
21–29	107	40.2	50.5	9.3
30–39	69	33.3	49.3	17.4
Over 39	56	41.1	51.8	7.1
Location				
London	79	49.4	41.8	8.9
Outside London	191	34.5	52.9	12.6

Note: [1] Figures for type of partner do not equal 270 as a few men who had both regular and casual partners are excluded.

Condom Use for Anal Intercourse

Among gay men one response to the threat of HIV has been to reduce the number of partners with whom they engage in anal intercourse (Joseph *et al.*, 1987; Evans *et al.*, 1989; Davies *et al.*, 1990). However, a significant proportion continue to engage in anal intercourse (Carne *et al.*, 1987; Fitzpatrick *et al.*, 1990; Hunt *et al.*, 1991). Since latex condoms have been proven capable of preventing the transmission of HIV *in vitro* and to reduce the risk of transmission *in vivo* (Conant *et al.*, 1986; Van de Perre, Jacobs and Sprecher-Goldberger, 1989), their uptake and continued use are of immense importance to the future spread of HIV infection.

Research in the United States (McKusick *et al.*, 1985, 1987; Martin, 1987; Fox *et al.*, 1987), Australia (Connell *et al.*, 1989; Gold *et al.*, 1989) and Europe (van Griensven *et al.*, 1989; Golombok, Sketchley and Rust, 1989; Weatherburn *et al.*, 1991) suggests that their widespread use has undoubtedly been a primary reason why earlier predictions of the course of the epidemic have proved to be over-estimates (Department of Health/Welsh Office, 1988). However, use is still far from universal. The following sections outline base rates of condom use and then examine some of the factors that affect their use.

We find that 29.0% (270) engaged in insertive anal intercourse, and 27.3% (n = 254) engaged in receptive anal intercourse in the month preceding interview. From Tables 9.7 and 9.8, which outline rates of condom use for these men, we see that aproximately 40% always use a condom, but nearly 50% never use one.

Factors Associated with Condom Use

As before, we consider the effects of geographical location, age group and type of sexual relationship on condom use. In addition the influence on condom use of

Table 9.8. Condom Use for Receptive Anal Intercourse (for those who engaged in anal intercourse in the last month)

	Total n	Always	Never (percentages)	Sometimes
All	254	42.5	45.7	11.8
Partner type[1]				
Regular	186	37.1	52.2	10.7
Casual	47	68.1	25.5	6.4
Relationship type				
Monogamous	80	33.8	55.0	11.2
Open	111	46.6	41.4	12.1
Age group				
<21	39	48.7	35.9	15.4
21–29	108	40.7	47.2	12.0
30–39	63	43.9	42.4	13.6
Over 39	41	39.0	56.1	4.9
Location				
London	85	50.6	41.2	8.2
Outside London	169	38.5	47.9	13.6

Note: [1] Figures for type of partner do not equal 254 as a few men who had both regular and casual partners are excluded.

other demographic, social and personality factors is assessed. In Tables 9.7 and 9.8, respectively, condom use figures are displayed broken down by type of relationship, type of sexual partner, geographical location and age group, for those who engaged in anal intercourse in the month before interview.

Sexual relationship status is the most significant factor in predicting condom use. This is true whether you consider condom use according to whether the partner is regular or casual and, for regular partners, whether that relationship is monogamous or open. For insertive anal intercourse (Table 9.7) 69.2% always used a condom with a casual compared with only 33.8% with a regular ($\chi^2 = 22.11$, df 2, $p < 0.001$). Similarly for receptive anal intercourse (Table 9.8) 68.1% always used with casuals compared with only 37.1% with regulars ($\chi^2 = 17.9$, df 2, $p < 0.001$). Condom use is significantly more likely with casual rather than regular partners.

Of the ninety-three respondents in a monogamous sexual relationship who had engaged in insertive anal intercourse in the preceding month, only 28% had always used a condom compared to 44.6% of those in open relationships ($\chi^2 = 7.1$, df 2, $p < 0.05$). The pattern is the same for receptive anal intercourse, although the result is not significant: 33.8% of those respondents in a monogamous relationship always use condoms compared to 46.6% for those in an open relationship ($\chi^2 = 4.65$, df 2, $p > 0.05$). Clearly, type of sexual partner is a significant predictor of condom use.

While not statistically significant, there are notable trends in condom usage by age groups. For insertive anal intercourse those respondents under the age of 21 are most likely always to use a condom and least likely never to do so. Those over 39 years of age were least likely always to use a condom and most likely never to use one. A similar pattern emerges for receptive anal intercourse. Of all the age groups, respondents under the age of 21 years are most likely always to use a condom, least likely never to use a condom. Those over 21 but under 39 are least likely always to use condoms and those over 39 are most likely never to use condoms.

While it is acknowledged that government health promotion activities, which were initiated in 1986, were equally accesible throughout England and Wales, it has been shown that changes in sexual behaviour not only predate these initiatives (Evans *et al.*, 1989) but are closely linked with voluntary sector and other targeted initiatives (Aggleton, Coxon and Weatherburn, 1990). These began far earlier, and are still more common and widespread within London. Thus for those who engage in anal intercourse the sample is subdivided into London (n = 120) and outside London (n = 263) in order to assess the impact of this differential availability of health promotion activities on unsafe sexual practices in general, and condom use in particular.

Our data reveal that those respondents in the London sample are significantly more likely always to use a condom (49.4% compared to 36.6%), and less likely never to use a condom (41.8% compared to 52.4%, $\chi^2 = 7.923$, df = 1, p. < 0.01) for insertive anal intercourse. While for receptive anal intercourse there are no significant results, the emergent trends are comparable. Clearly, and as predicted, condom use for anal intercourse is more widespread and consistent within the capital than outside.

The analysis thus far reports only two-way associations. A log-linear analysis indicates no interaction effects (that is, no higher order associations) for condom use for either insertive or receptive anal intercourse.[1] For the models chosen the co-efficient of multiple determination is 0.91 for insertive and 0.90 for receptive anal intercourse. Thus the two-way associations identified in the preceding sections account for 90% of the variation in the condom use data.

None of the following demographic variables significantly distinguished between respondents who always used condoms and those who did not, among those who engaged in anal intercourse in the month preceding interview: highest educational qualification; social class; political affiliation; religious affiliation; religious interest. Similarly none of the following gay identification and integration factors predicted condom use: homosexual regret; degree of disclosure; degree to which respondents wished they had been born heterosexual; degree to which respondents wished they could henceforth be heterosexual; self-assessed sexual appeal to other men; self-identified sexual feelings and sexual behaviour; whether or not respondents had ever seriously considered discontinuing their gay activities; and whether or not they had ever sought professional advice concerning their sexuality.

A range of factors pertaining to HIV/AIDS was also of no predictive value. These included: knowledge of HIV transmission routes; knowledge of safer sex recommendations regarding condoms, and having taken the HIV test. Finally, a range of personality factors was found not to predict condom using behaviour, including: a self-reported suicide attempt; self-rated depression, anxiety and self-conciousness; self-efficacy; and sexual communication skills.

Of all the factors examined very few are significantly associated with condom use. Those that are are outlined below, as they may prove instructive. There is a significant association between condom use for receptive anal intercourse and number of male partners in the last month ($F = 9.7$, df = 1, $p < .01$). The respondents who always used a condom for being fucked had a significantly greater mean number of male partners (3.6 against 2.1). There are no significant relationships between condom use for insertive anal intercourse and numbers of partners in the last month. However, there is no significant association between condom use for either insertive or receptive anal intercourse and *number of penetrative sexual partners*. Clearly, conclusions regarding condom use that rely upon examination of absolute partner numbers alone should be treated with caution, as any proclaimed causal links may be spurious.

Marital status is significantly related to condom use for insertive (but not receptive) anal intercourse ($\chi^2 = 6.27$, df = 2, p. < .05). Those men who are married (or cohabiting with a female) are significantly more likely always to use a condom for insertive anal intercourse (75% compared to 34.7% of singles and 45.8% who are divorced, widowed or separated). This lends support to the argument (Boulton *et al.*, 1990) that behaviourally bisexual males are more likely to engage in safer sexual practices with men than exclusively homosexual men. Of note is the fact that of those respondents who had engaged in vaginal intercourse in the month preceding interview 54% never used a condom, 28% always did and 18% sometimes used one.

Perceived HIV status is also associated with condom use for insertive anal intercourse ($\chi^2 = 6.46$, df = 1, p. < .01). Those respondents who believe, suspect or know themselves to be HIV antibody positive are significantly more likely always to use a condom (56.5%) than respondents who believe, suspect or know themselves to be HIV antibody negative (34.3%). This suggests that those respondents who perceive themselves to be HIV antibody postive are better at protecting their partners than those who perceive themselves to be antibody negative are at protecting themselves.

The final variable significantly associated with condom use is the response to the question, '*How seriously do you take safer sex*?' Of those respondents who answered 'not at all', 'not very' or 'moderately', only 13.5% always used a condom for insertive anal intercourse. Conversely, of those who answered 'very' or 'very indeed', 43.1% always used a condom, and of those who answered 'extremely', 43.5% always did ($\chi^2 = 15.74$, df = 2, p. < .001). For receptive anal intercourse of those answering 'not at all', 'not very' or 'moderately', only 22.9% always used a condom. Of those who answered 'very' or 'very indeed', 45.8% always used a condom, and of those who answered 'extremely', 50.6% always did ($\chi^2 = 10.20$, df = 2, p. < .001). While the relationship between this variable and condom using behaviour (and engagement in anal intercourse) is neither surprising nor particularly illuminating, it does confirm that self-reported attitudinal measures can be usefully compared to current sexual behaviour.

Major Implications

To plan effectively and implement future health education initiatives, it is essential to understand why some men never use condoms even though they continue to engage in anal intercourse. While the vast majority know that using condoms for anal intercourse reduces the risk of HIV transmission, less than half always used a condom for anal intercourse.

While condoms are used relatively consistently with casual partners, unprotected anal intercourse is common in regular relationships, particularly those characterised by love and trust. Given that asymptomatic HIV infection can last as long as ten years and the mean relationship lifespan within this cohort is four years (Davies *et al.*, 1990: 96), the non-use of condoms within relationships is not necessarily a safe strategy, especially if, as has been argued (Prieur, 1990: Gold *et al.*, 1989), condoms are often discarded relatively early in the course of a relationship as a sign of mutual trust and commitment. Thus the need to use a condom even in a long-term relationship should be made clear in all health education initiatives (see also Chapter 11).

A greater proportion of men under the age of 21 always use a condom for anal intercourse and a smaller proportion never use a condom. Given the widespread belief that young gay men are at greater risk of HIV infection, these results are especially important. These data may be interpreted as indicating an emergent culture of condom use among the men under 21. They have become sexually active since HIV/AIDS, and the recent growth in popularity of condoms coupled with a relaxation of associated stigma may have made their use more normative. However, given that they are more sexually active and more likely to be engaging in anal intercourse, it is particularly important that their condom use is continually reinforced; though given that their behaviour is illegal, this may be particularly problematic.

Older men — especially those who were sexually active before the liberalisation of the law in 1967, and long before the advent of HIV/AIDS — seem less inclined to adopt advice on health protective behavioural changes. This may be because anal intercourse had been central to their sexual repertoire or perhaps because of their age they are simply less open to change in general. Whatever the reason specific emphasis should be put on targeting the older generation for advice on condom use.

Finally, it is interesting to note that within the UK there are significant variations in condom use by geographical location. For insertive anal intercourse a significantly greater proportion of the London cohort always use a condom, in comparison with outside London. This effect is noticeable across all sexual relationship types and all age groups. Most health education initiatives targeted at homosexually active males have emanated from London (Aggleton, Coxon and Weatherburn, 1990) where specific advice for gay men has been, and to some extent still is, more widely available. By contrast, homosexually active males outside London only have access to national campaigns which are more vague and certainly less salient with regard to their sexual behaviour. Clearly, health educators should consider targeted campaigns outside London.

Sexual Behaviour with Women

Men who have sex with both men and women are often seen as crucial to the pattern of sexual spread of HIV and the future incidence of AIDS (Winkelstein *et al.*, 1986; Bennett *et al.*, 1989; Ekstrand *et al.*, 1992). In this context it is rarely acknowledged that self-avowed sexual identity is of relatively little consequence; or that there is no straightforward relationship between self-proclaimed sexual identity and sexual behaviour (Boulton and Weatherburn, 1990; Fitzpatrick *et al.*, 1989; Weatherburn *et al.*, 1990).

Hence we not only have to recognise the possibility of the existence of bisexual men who are attracted to and sexually active with both males and females,

Table 9.9. Sexual Activity with Women (percentages)

Sexual act	Ever	Current
Deep Kissing	55.5	4.0
Vaginal intercourse	51.8	4.8
Masturbation	41.5	4.5
Oral sex	38.7	4.0
Massage	26.3	2.4
Body rubbing	25.5	3.1
Anal fingering	13.4	1.5
Inter-femoral	12.7	0.5
Anal intercourse	9.7	0.3
Anilingus	5.2	0.5

but we have to recognise that some 'heterosexual' men have sex with other men, and that being gay does not necessarily mean you never have sexual contact with women. In terms of HIV what is at issue is not sexual identity, but the specific pattern of sexual activity, particularly the prevalence of those acts most likely to be implicated in the spread of the HIV: vaginal and anal intercourse (Padian *et al.*, 1987; Johnson and Laga, 1988).

As Table 9.9 illustrates, during the course of their lives over half of this cohort of predominantly gay men has had vaginal intercourse. Furthermore, about 40% have engaged in masturbation with a female, and a similar proportion in oral sex. Finally, about one-quarter have massaged and body rubbed, and one-eighth have anally fingered or had inter-crural intercourse with a female.

Data on the prevalence of other sexual acts with a female, are briefly outlined to demonstrate the diversity of heterosexual behaviour among these men. Given the dearth of comparable data, it is impossible to make comparisons with exclusively heterosexual dyads (but see Boulton *et al.*, 1990). However, it is interesting to note that with an incidence of just under 10%, anal intercourse is not significantly more common within these sexual relationships than for exclusively heterosexual couples (Evans *et al.*, 1988), and may indeed be less so (Fulford *et al.*, 1983).

In the preceding month the percentage of respondents engaging in each act with a female was relatively small: for example, 4.5% had masturbated with a female in the preceding month in comparison with nearly 75% who had masturbated with a male in the same period. Just over 4% of the cohort had had oral sex with a female in the preceding month, and, although 9.7% of respondents claimed to have ever had anal sex with a female, only three had done so in the month preceding interview.

In terms of HIV transmission it is important to note that vaginal intercourse is not only the sexual act with the highest prevalence but also at 4.8% it is the act with the highest current incidence. Of those men who reported currently engaging in vaginal intercourse 53% (n = 23) never used a condom, 28% (n = 12) always did and 19% (n = 8) sometimes used one (data not available for two respondents).

Current 'Behavioural Bisexuality'

In the year before interview 9.3% had had sexual contact with both males and females and just 2.5% had sex only with females. This corresponds fairly closely with both the self-reported Kinsey ratings of the cohort, in which just over 90% identified themselves as either exclusively or predominantly gay, and with other research (Fitzpatrick *et al.*, 1990).

In terms of HIV transmission it is vitally important to note that during the previous year the proportion of men having *penetrative* sex with both males and females is smaller than the 9.3% outlined above. Thus in the preceding year 6.3% had engaged in both anal intercourse with a male and vaginal intercourse with a female, and in the preceding month 0.65% (n = 6) reported having engaged in anal intercourse with a male and vaginal intercourse with a female. In the month preceding interview none of the respondents had engaged in anal intercourse with both a male and a female.

While it would be foolhardy to attempt to draw any firm conclusions from such small numbers, it is interesting to note that of the six respondents who had penetrative sex with both males and females in the month preceding interview, only one always used a condom with all penetrative partners, although four always used a condom for insertive anal intercourse with a male. The other two always used a condom for vaginal intercourse, but never or only sometimes used one for insertive anal intercourse.

Finally, those who currently have sex with both males and females appear to be significantly younger than the rest ($\chi^2 = 6.416$, df = 2, p = < .05). This may be explained by the observation that men at the start of their sexual careers are more likely to experiment with partners of both sexes. Apart from Kinsey self-ratings, no other factors were significantly related to 'behavioural bisexuality'.

Sexual Partners

Epidemiologists and sexual athletes are interested in gross estimates of partner numbers, if for different reasons. While the focus of epidemiological attention is on the estimation of the rate of spread of HIV, the interest of the athletes lies in the number of men to be captured in order to make in into the record books. It turns out, however, that what people mean when they use the term 'sexual partner' differs widely, so the aims of both groups may need to be reassessed.

What Is a Sexual Partner?

Early in the research it became clear that the terms 'sexual encounter' and 'a sexual partner' are ambiguous. Many research studies naively ask gay and bisexual men, 'How many sexual partners have you had in the last month/year/ten years?', and make two crucial assumptions: first, that all men count the same behaviours as marking a sexual encounter; and second, that this figure could be regarded as a valid measure of risk with respect to HIV transmission. Neither of these assumptions is correct (Hunt and Davies, 1990). We asked the men in the cohort: 'Suppose someone asked you "How many sexual partners have you had this month?", what must have happened sexually for someone to "count" as your sexual partner?' Table 9.10 shows the main categories emerging in answer to this question. Broadly speaking, the responses fall into one of two groups: either physical (that is, pertaining to some form of actual physical contact) or affective (that is, descriptions

Table 9.10. Counts of Categories Noted When Asked to Define a Sexual Partner (percentages[1])

Genital contact of which:	48
Penetration[2]	6
Anal sex	5
Orgasm	26
Bed/Naked/Sleep with	22
Physical contact	7
Eroticism/Arousal	3
Aim for orgasm	2
See more than once	2
Privacy	<1

Notes: [1] Some mentioned more than one category so percentage total >100.
[2] Penetration includes both oral and anal sex.

which are highly contextual or which refer to emotional states) in a ratio of about three to one. We concluded that the term 'sexual partner' had two distinct meanings: either simply someone with whom some form of sex occurred, or someone with whom 'special' sex occurred, that is, sex with some emotional charge. There were no differences by age (t statistic = 0.098, p = 0.46) or relationship type ($\chi^2 = 2.574$, df 2, p = 0.28). Since only 5% indicated that anal intercourse was the important marker of a sexual encounter, and given our finding that the staples of the sexual repertoire are acts which are safe with respect to HIV transmission, then using measures of partner numbers as indicators of HIV risk appears to be misguided.

'Sexual Partners' and Epidemiology

Nevertheless, it is important to gain some understanding of the impact of partner numbers on HIV risk, so during the interview respondents were introduced to a standard definition of sexual partner: 'A sexual partner is any person with whom you have had sexual contact, where the aim was orgasm for one or both of you.' There remain a few problems with this definition, mainly concerning the meaning of the term 'sexual' which we took to mean 'physical, genital contact'. It also excludes some activities such as voyeuristic sex, the use of telephone sex lines and some sado-masochistic activities. It should be noted that some of these non-physical forms of sexual expression have probably increased in popularity in recent years due, at least in part, to their safety with respect to HIV transmission. This omission seemed a reasonable restriction, however, given our prime interest in the transmission of HIV.

In addition, a penetrative sexual partner (or, as it became known, a 'PSP') was defined as 'a sexual partner whom you fucked (either anally or vaginally) or who fucked you.' Concentrating on PSPs carries a number of advantages:

since numbers of PSPs are lower than number of partners and the significance of anal intercourse is greater than other kinds of sex, it is likely that these estimates will be more accurate;

numbers of PSPs give a more accurate parameter for epidemiological predictions of spread of HIV than numbers of partners;

Table 9.11. Distribution of the Reported Numbers of Male Sexual Partners and PSPs in Lifetime, Five Years, Year and Month Before First Interview (1987–88)

Partners			PSPs
	Lifetime		
Number	%	Number	%
0	2.6	0	8.9
1	1.3	1	8.6
2–10	19.6	2–10	42.6
11–50	35.0	11–50	23.6
51–100	11.1	51–100	6.6
101–500	21.2	101–500	7.1
501–1000	3.3	501–1000	1.6
>1000	5.8	>1000	1.0
	Past five years		
Number	%	Number	%
0	3.2	0	14.2
1	3.8	1	15.1
2–10	34.7	2	12.7
11–50	38.8	3	11.0
51–100	8.3	4	7.8
101–200	6.0	5	5.3
>200	5.2	6–10	14.4
		11–50	15.1
		>50	4.4
	Last year		
Number	%	Number	%
0	6.3	0	30.9
1	14.6	1	31.2
2–10	56.2	2–10	34.5
11–50	20.1	11–50	3.3
>50	2.8	>50	0.1
	Last month		
Number	%	Number	%
0	23.4	0	59.7
1	39.3	1	31.6
2	15.6	2	6.2
3–5	15.2	>2	2.5
>5	6.5		

coincidentally, it enables us to make more meaningful comparisons with other studies, particularly those of heterosexual behaviour, where partners are usually assumed to be synonymous with PSPs.

Numbers of Sexual Partners

Tables 9.11 and 9.12 present the numbers of male sexual partners and PSPs for the lifetime and for the five years, year and month prior to the first interview

Table 9.12. Summary Statistics for Reported Numbers of Male Partners and PSPs at Wave one (1987–88)

	Partners			
	Lifetime	Five years	Last year	Last month
Median	38	16	4	1
Lower quartile	12	5	2	1
Upper quartile	181	40	10	2
Mean	279	52	11	2
Standard deviation	1101	126	22	3
Maximum	25000	1500	300	40
	Penetrative sexual partners			
	Lifetime	Five years	Last year	Last month
Median	7	3	1	0
Lower quartile	2	1	0	0
Upper quartile	25	9	2	1
Mean	79	12	2	1
Standard deviation	459	36	5	1
Maximum	1000	750	70	15

(1987–88). It is important to note that all the distributions considered are skewed towards the smaller numbers. There is a very small number of men who have considerably higher numbers of sexual partners than the vast majority of the cohort. This affects the mean measure considerably, and thus our preferred measure of level is the median. These figures illustrate that the number of partners and PSPs gay men have varies enormously. In any given period some have very many, some very few, and others have none at all. At wave one a very small proportion of men (< 3%) reported never having had a male sexual partner but remained in the study on the basis that they are attracted to men and/or identify as gay. A larger proportion (9%) reported never having had a male penetrative sexual partner (PSP).

For the Five Years from 1982 to 1987

The period between 1982 and 1987 was one in which HIV and AIDS came to prominence, and numbers of partners and PSPs from this period may reflect the effect of gay community campaigns promoting safer sexual practices.

4% reported no sexual partners;
the median number of partners is sixteen;
half the men reported between five and forty partners;
16% reported no PSPs;
the median number of PSPs in three;
half reported between one and nine.

In the year before the first interview:

6% reported no sexual partners;
the median number of partners is four;
half of the men reported between two and ten partners;
less than 10% reported more than twenty-six partners;
31% reported no PSPs;
the median number of PSPs is one;
half of the men reported between none and two PSPs;
less than 10% reported more than four PSPs.

In the month before the first interview:

23% reported no partners;
the median number of partners is one;
half of the men reported either one or two partners;
Nearly 95% reported fewer than five partners;
60% reported no PSPs;
the median number of PSPs is none;
over 90% reported either one or no PSPs.

Although numbers of partners are always higher than numbers of PSPs, the relationship between the two is not consistent (Hunt *et al.*, 1991). In the last year the mean proportion of partners who are penetrative is 36.7% and the median is 25%. On either measure the incidence of penetrative partners is lower than might be assumed from applying heterosexual assumptions to homosexual behaviour. The crucial questions for epidemiologists are, however: (1) whether the proportion of partners who are penetrative remains stable as the numbers of partners rise; and (2) whether the proportion is stable over time.

To test this, the ratio of PSPs to partners for groups of partners (grouped in steps of ten partners) has been investigated. Analysis of variance reveals significant differences between the ratios for each group ($F_{6,864} = 12.839$, $p < 0.001$) with the ratio being the highest for the group with less than ten partners and lowest for the groups above this level. Furthermore, even though the data below ten partners may be consistent with the view that the proportion of PSPs is constant, the figure reveals a wide variation around the mean, rendering the relationship of limited use for modelling purposes. The low correlation coefficient ($r^2 = 0.04$) confirms the lack of any relationship. Thus rate of partner change combined with infectivity measures are unreliable in estimating risks of HIV infection.

Female Partners

In their lifetime over 60% of respondents reported having had sexual contact with a female and 50% reported a female PSP. Considering the entire cohort, 60.6% (562) reported having had sexual contact with a female in their lifetime and 52.5% (448) reported at least one penetrative female partner. The median lifetime number is one partner and one penetrative sexual partner. In the last five years over 30% reported a female partner and 27% reported a female PSP. In the five years before wave one just under a third reported a female partner and about the same proportion reported a penetrative sexual partner (PSP). The median number for female partners and female PSPs is none in the last year (means 0.47 and 0.22 respectively). In the last year 12% reported a female partner and 11% reported a female PSP. In the year before interview 11.7% (109) reported a female partner and 10.6% (99) reported a penetrative female partner. In the preceding month 5% reported a female partner and 5% reported a female PSP. In the month before interview 5.4% (50) males reported a female partner, of which 4.8% (45) were penetrative. No respondent reported more than three female partners in the month prior to interview.

Among those males who have had sex with males and females in any time period, the average number of female partners is significantly lower than the number of male partners. However, the proportion of female partners with whom penetration occurs is very much higher than for male partners. For all the time periods considered, the mean proportion of female partners which are penetrative never falls below 0.81, whereas for male partners the mean ratio never exceeds 0.40. Clearly, epidemiological models need to take account of the proportion of partnerships in which penile penetration occurs, rather than rates of partner change alone.

Factors Affecting Partner Numbers

The only factors that significantly affect partner numbers are age, geographic location and whether respondents had been HIV tested. Obviously, older men in the cohort will have had more lifetime partners and PSPs than younger men, but there is no evidence to suggest that they were any more or less sexually active in their earlier years than younger men are today. However, older men tend to have fewer current partners and significantly fewer of these are PSPs. Men living in London have higher numbers of partners and PSPs, but outside the capital a greater proportion of partners are penetrative. Men who had taken an HIV antibody test were likely to have more partners and PSPs.

Note

1 The application of log-linear models to social sciences was developed and explained in Gilbert (1982). The method provides a way of assessing orders of association in multivariate contingency tables.

10 Perspectives on Fucking

'even identical genital acts mean very different things to different people'.
Eve Kosofsky-Sedgewick (1991: 16)

In the previous chapter we have seen how diverse is the sexual experience of the men in the cohort. In particular, we have drawn attention to the fact that anal intercourse plays an important part in the sexual repertoire of many gay men. In the next chapter we describe the ways in which the dangers associated with anal intercourse in the time of HIV are managed by these men, both individually and in negotiation. Given the immense symbolic significance of anal intercourse and its pivotal role in the transmission of HIV, however, we devote this chapter to an examination of the different meanings that men ascribe to anal intercourse. Central to this discussion is the conviction that anal intercourse is not something men *must* do (and cannot help themselves from doing), but something they actively *choose* to do in some circumstances and not in others.

Male Homosexuality and Anal Intercourse

Social sanction against the anal penetration of the male body seems to have characterised Western civilisation since at least the classical period. Despite widespread and socially acceptable sexual encounters between young men and boys, anal penetration, especially of adult free males, was frowned upon. The tract *Against Timarchus* (discussed by Foucault, 1985: 215ff.), argues the incompatibility of citizenship with the enjoyment of anal intercourse. Because the male body stood as a metaphor for the state, its inviolability was a metaphoric bulwark against invasion. By allowing penetration, the citizen gave up his claim to be a 'real' man and thus, argues Aeschines, should forego the privileges of citizenship.

The confinement of disapproval to the 'passive' partner in anal intercourse — to the one who is penetrated — while other forms of homosexual expression, even the 'active' role, are either sanctioned or condoned, remains a feature of many contemporary societies, particularly those with their cultural origins in the Mediterranean. Such a pattern has been described in Nicaragua, where a man who allows himself to be penetrated is termed a *cochón* (Lancaster, 1988), in Mexico (Carrier, 1971, 1976) in the construction of the Brazilian *bicha* (Young, 1973) as well as contemporary Turkey (Tapinc, 1992) and elsewhere (Murray, 1992). In a very real sense the male who allows himself to be penetrated in these cultures represents a separate gender: that of feminine male.

Medieval scholasticism condemned all sexual expression outside marriage, yet recognised, following Aquinas, a gradation of sin. His category of 'unnatural sin' includes, in increasing order of sinfulness: masturbation, least sinful because it involves no other person; lechery, which 'involves improper manners of intercourse, and this is worse if it is not effected in the proper vessel than if the perversion of the sex act is done in some other way'; sodomy, because the wrong sex is involved; and, finally, bestiality, because it crosses the species barrier. Gradually, all sexual transgressions, including anal intercourse between men, became subsumed under the term 'sodomy'. The usage continued into the early modern period. Gilbert (1981) claims anal intercourse, irrespective of the gender of the partner, has always been castigated to a greater extent. Huusen (1989: 145) has suggested that the death penalty was reserved for sodomy only when anal penetration could be proven.

In the late nineteenth century researchers and writers such as Edward Carpenter and Havelock Ellis, while asking for understanding and tolerance of homosexuality, were at pains to point out that the condition did not automatically involve anal intercourse; and despite the fact that this contention has been repeated in most texts on male homosexuality since (for example, Westwood, 1960; Schofield, 1965a: 35; Kinsey, 1948), the message seems not to have been heard.

In Nazi concentration camps, before the pink triangle was used to designate those convicted under Paragraph 175 (homosexual offences), a yellow stripe inscribed with a large black 'A' was used, designating the wearer as an *Arschficker* (arse-fucker) (Haeberle, 1981). During the debate over the 1967 Sexual Offences Act, the campaigner Antony Grey claimed (Jeffrey-Poulter, 1991: 87) that he could no longer bear them 'burbling on about buggery'. Indeed, the 1967 Bill was dubbed 'the bugger's charter', although it does not specifically refer to anal intercourse. Little has changed. When the infamous Clause 28 of the 1988 Local Government Act was being debated in the House of Commons (see Chapter 3), Mrs Kellett-Bowman (member for Lancaster), in reply to whether 'Other people's [i.e., homosexual] relationships should be accepted by all civilised adults', stated: 'It depends on what one means by "civilised". I do not regard the practice of sodomy or buggery as being civilised' (*Hansard*, 15 December 1987). Here, with no justification, she equates homosexuality with 'sodomy or buggery'. It is unlikely that she was aware of the archaic meaning of sodomy (see below), and it is almost certain that she was not thinking of lesbianism when she said it.

With the advent of the modern gay liberation movement, particularly the Gay Liberation Fronts of the early 1970s, fucking took on a political meaning, as people started challenging the traditional roles and positions of men and women. Fucking became a two-fingered salute to the established order and conventional morality. A Parisian Front Homosexual Action Révolutionnaire leaflet stated: 'we get fucked by Arabs. We're proud of it and will do it again. . . . Our asshole is revolutionary' (Adam, 1987: 87). For many gay men, receptive fucking became a liberating experience, a release from stifling gender boundaries, that demanded they always be initiatory, active and penetrators. By claiming men can be fucked, and that they can enjoy it, was to call into question the fixedness of what it meant to be 'a man'.

On the other hand, there were those in the movement who regarded anal intercourse as aping and perpetuating oppressive heterosexually-based norms. These included those who were influenced by feminist theory and also Larry Kramer (1978) who pleaded, 'why do faggots fuck so fucking much?' It would seem, however, that he was despairing about a particular milieu of 'fast lane' New York gay men. Carrier (1977) suggests that the extent of anal fucking within a homosexual population is associated with how strongly the distinction between masculinity and femininity is made within the population as a whole. This in turn is related to whether homosexually active men develop sex role preferences (that is, a butch/femme model). He states that 'in the societies where the majority of the homosexually involved males appear to develop sex-role preferences, anal fucking is preferred over fellatio.' Conversely, in populations where there is less sex-role playing, as in Anglo-American samples, fellatio is more common.

Gay men are typically reviled for their presumed practice of anal intercourse. Jokes at the expense of gay men invariably revolve around fucking, and the gamut of derogatory terms usually play on that act ('dirt box snatcher', 'sausage jokey', 'uphill gardener', 'shit stabber', 'chocolate box poker', 'brown hatter'). The oft-heard cry of straight men when encountering gay men, 'Backs against the wall lads!', also implies that their rears are the only thing gay men would be interested in, while simultaneously revealing their dread fear of being penetrated.

Morin (1986: 20–1) gives a four-fold reason for the taboo on anal sexuality in his ground-breaking book, *Anal Pleasure and Health*. The first concerns the general association of the anus with uncleanliness: 'by becoming symbolic of all that is unclean, and fostering the emotion of disgust, the anus and faeces serve to focus and intensify the value placed on being clean.' He proposes that 'the anal taboo expresses and perpetuates a more general mistrust of the body, it makes concrete the conflict between spirit and body, increases guilt, and thereby reinforces religious doctrine.' Third, and most pertinently here, 'another possible function of the anal taboo is the maintenance of strict sex-role differentiation.' Morin suggests that the general taboo on anal sexuality has the more focused intention of preventing men from being anally penetrated, and 'all that it symbolizes' (although he doesn't go into detail about what it does symbolise). The fourth and related function 'is to bolster sanctions against homosexual behaviour, particularly among men.'

Michel Foucault (1982/3: 21) has hypothesised that this reticence stems from presumed changes in the image men believe women hold of them when being receptive. All men, he says, including homosexual men, 'think of themselves as existing in the minds of women as masters' and that 'the idea of their submitting to another man . . . would destroy their image in the eyes of women.' He concludes that 'today homosexuals still have this problem. Most homosexuals feel that the passive role is in some way demeaning.' Why it should be the destruction of women's presumed image, rather than the image presumed to be held by other men, is not explained. It seems to us more likely that the fear of being receptive stems from danger to the regard one is held in by other men (especially the insertive partner), or to the regard one holds oneself in (one's self-image). Being receptive is associated with being not wholly 'masculine', or in being identified as a woman in some way. In a culture such as our own, in which it is insulting to call a male 'a woman', and any male who gives up the power involved in being 'a man' is to be ridiculed, being fucked can be problematic. One way of dealing with this problem is to reject the implicit values of a patriarchal culture.

To many people, both gay and straight, fucking is often seen as a wilful perversity. If it is not seen as perverse, it never gains meaning beyond the purely physical. This may be part of a larger prejudice that follows the logic that many gay men have anonymous casual sex with no emotional commitment, therefore all homosexual sex is purely physical with no emotional loading. The deployment of HIV education messages carries the implicit assumption that the physical pleasures of fucking can be replaced with other sexual acts. The 'eroticising' of safer sex ignores any difference of meaning of fucking from other acts. This assumption is based on a double-pronged prejudice: that gay sex is first and foremost grounded in physical pleasure, and participation in it is just something to do, a hobby, like stamp collecting; second, that the focus of the hobby can be changed with ease.

Even ten years into the HIV epidemic there is a dearth of work on how fucking fits into gay men's lives and relationships. One of the few exceptions is the work of Prieur (1990), who identified reasons for unprotected fucking in terms of a lack of social support, and of sexual behaviour as a set of communicative acts. She claimed that her Norwegian respondents who had had unprotected fucking used sex as a primary means of achieving closeness. Safer sex was associated with death and distrust, and experienced as emotionally cold. She goes further in identifying orgasm during fucking, and the receiving of semen into the anus, as an act of commitment to the partner. Whether or not these understandings can be generalised to gay men outside Norway (or even outside Oslo) is debatable. She does, however, ground sexual behaviour in a language of love and affection, which is conspicuously absent from other commentaries. In the next part of this chapter we examine the complex and disparate understandings, feelings and attitudes that the men in our cohort had about anal intercourse.

What Gay Men Think and Feel about Fucking

In wave four of Project SIGMA, men were asked: 'How important is fucking to you?' This introductory question was followed by the question: 'Why is it important/not important?', and the men were encouraged to talk freely about their perceptions and experiences. The only further two prompts used were: 'Tell me about the difference between active and passive fucking?' and 'What differences has HIV made?' Men were also asked whether they agreed or disagreed with twenty-nine statements about fucking. Agreement or disagreement was then examined in relation to whether or not the respondent had fucked or been fucked, with regular and casual partners in the last year. What the men said in the open-ended part of the interview was organised by themes. These themes are not mutually exclusive and often overlap. Most converge when the men talk about fucking with regular partners versus casual partners, and this theme is left until last, although it is mentioned in some of the preceding themes.

Centrality

The first responses to the question, 'How important is fucking to you?', were usually a general assessment of the centrality of fucking to their sexual and social lives. As we shall see later, this centrality marker is not static throughout a person's life, and is rarely constant between different sexual partners or even sessions. That is, it may be very important to fuck in a particular session with a particular partner, and unimportant or undesirable in another session with the same or different partner. As one respondent put it, 'It depends: sometimes it's very important, sometimes not at all.' However, all the men made an initial assessment (whether or not later qualified). These were grouped into three categories.

1 Fucking as primary, central, very or quite important to sexual life: 46.6% of responses were classified in this group. Responses included: 'Very important' (n = 55); 'Quite important' (n = 31); 'Important' (n = 23); 'It is an important part of sex for me. If we didn't fuck, sex would be missing something.' 'It's essential. It's a need, its not an option.'
2 Fucking as coincidental, of secondary or minor importance: 34.5% of responses including: 'Not very important' (n = 47); 'Not that important' (n = 19); 'Not particularly important' (n = 10); 'I suppose I could live without it if I had to, but it's a pleasure.' 'It's just one thing to do of many.'
3 Fucking as of no importance, or having overall negative qualities: 18.9% of responses including: 'Not at all important' (n = 28); 'Not important' (n = 24); 'Absolutely doesn't feature in things. I'm 47 and I cannot for the life of me imagine how someone can have a cock shoved up their arse.' 'It's just never been part of my sex life, and even when I had a long term affair in the 1970s it was rare that we screwed together.'

The centrality of fucking to one's sex life is a very gross measure and does not indicate whether it will feature in a particular sexual session. A man may think fucking was absolutely essential, but if the person he is having sex with hates it, it probably will not occur. Although a large proportion fall into category 1 above, this does not mean they engage in fucking, or would wish to, in every sexual session they are involved in: 'I couldn't live without it, not completely, even though I don't fuck often.' The desirability of fucking in any one session is dependent on a large number of things. Some of these are individual (how turned on you are by the general idea, if you find it painful or not), some are interpersonal (how attractive you find your partner, whether you trust him), and some are situational (whether a condom is available, whether sex is likely to be interrupted).

Agreement or disagreement with the two statements that looked at centrality are both significantly predictive of whether individuals had fucked in the last year for both modalities and both partner types. For example, of those who agreed with 'I can't imagine giving up fucking indefinitely', 47% had fucked a casual partner compared to 25% of those who disagreed with the statement ($\chi^2 = 21.54$, df = 2, $p < 0.0001$). Similarly, 40% of those who agreed with 'Fucking is *not* an essential part of my sex life' had been fucked by a regular partner, but 59% of those disagreeing had ($\chi^2 = 17.41$, df = 2, $p < 0.0001$).

Identity (n = 11)

Few men mentioned gay identity aspects of fucking, but their reports are included here as gay community involvement and positive self-image have been proposed as important correlates in sexual behaviour (Weinberg, 1978; Connell *et al.*, 1989; Bochow, 1990; Soskolne *et al.*, 1991; Kippax *et al.*, 1992). Those who did mention identity bear witness to the variability of understandings. Some men reported fucking, especially being fucked, as reinforcing their sense of being a gay man: 'There's a political element, part of my identity as gay man.' 'Being fucked makes me feel more gay and that's something I like.' Other men felt oppressed by the cultural coupling of male homosexuality and fucking, and resisted it: 'I resent the assumption that all gay people do that.' 'I've got the feeling that a great many people feel it's the prime thing done by gay people, my own experience in the gay world is that a great many don't engage in penetrative sex.'

There is evidence here of the fluidity of understandings over time. One's experience of fucking can change over the course of a sexual career: 'It was just something that never appealed to me, I hated the label of "homosexual" meaning putting your cock up someone's bum or vice versa. Now a lot of it is about letting myself go, I'm coming along as a gay man.' Interestingly, two men talked about the sex they had had with men who did not identify as gay. They gave complementary yet contradictory accounts of the role of fucking in these encounters: 'My partners haven't been into fucking in the recent past. It's to do with them not feeling gay and not wanting to explore that side of themselves.' 'In the sessions where I was active the men were straight, they more or less wanted to explore the sensation of being fucked.'

Further insight into the way some men conceptualise the link between being gay and fucking can be gleaned from what was said about sex with women. Some men felt fucking to be in some way mimicking heterosexual sex, and this to be a good reason to avoid it: 'It's [fucking] too much like married life . . . in married life you fuck, I've opted out of married life into gay life.' 'It's not physical revulsion, something psychological about it, penetration is too heterosexual for me.' Others, however, made the parallel between fucking and heterosexuality, but did not view it as problematic: 'I feel the same as a fellow would towards a girl. I don't see how you can differentiate between gay sex and heterosexual activity, the ultimate with a guy or a girl is to screw, I don't see why gays should feel any different about it.' Fucking was by no means always seen as normative. The appeal for some men lay in its transgression of 'acceptable behaviour': 'Naughtiness comes to mind, it flies in the face of that part of me that feels I shouldn't.' 'I like the idea because it's something you shouldn't really do, it's forbidden, not really socially acceptable.' However, this would appear to be a minority view since only 14% agreed that 'Fucking is a rebellious act', only 3% agreeing strongly. Thus fucking does not have one true meaning, and can at once be normative and transgressive.

Physical Pleasure (n = 63)

The contention that gay men fuck because it feels good is supported. It would be surprising if large numbers of men claimed it to be physically unpleasant but did it anyway. Physical feeling was explicitly mentioned by sixty-three men: 'It's a lovely feeling. I really can't expand on that, it's truly wonderful.' 'It's just a sensation I don't get any other way, that's true for active and passive.' Pleasurable sensations were mentioned equally in the contexts of being insertive and receptive: 'Mainly it's for physical pleasure as I really enjoy the sensation of fucking someone.'

'I enjoy being penetrated, the sensation. If I felt I had to give up being fucked I would have to use dildoes.'

Although physical pleasure was mentioned by many men, 25% agreed and only 11% strongly agreed with 'Fucking is the *most* pleasurable form of sex.' Other types of sex were often cited as being more pleasurable: 'If I have to choose between oral sex and anal sex I'd take oral every time — I'm a slut and just love licking and sucking. If I see a big cock my first instinct is to suck it.' 'Since having long term, more regular partners affection has taken over, I prefer a good cuddle as opposed to a good fuck.'

Orgasm (n = 39)

Linked to physical pleasure is the orgasm achieved through fucking. The thirty-nine men who mentioned orgasms varied in how they thought they were related to fucking. Some considered it gave them the best orgasms when being insertive: 'It's in the mind, more intense orgasm than by any other means.' 'Fucking someone is the most satisfying way to have orgasm and that's physiological.' Being fucked can also encourage a more intense orgasm: 'Coming with someone inside me is more powerful.' Having an orgasm merely by being fucked was occasionally mentioned: 'The main object is for me to relax and ejaculate when being screwed without being touched by hand.' 'I can come [when being fucked] if it's done right, stimulated to coming and I don't need to wank.' Better orgasm through fucking was certainly not everyone's experience. For some, other forms of sex were more instrumental: 'I've had much better orgasms with a wank, but I still enjoy fucking.' For a few, fucking was merely a route to orgasm with no other meaning: 'Having an orgasm is having an orgasm. The act itself doesn't do anything for me.' Or it was not a route to orgasm at all: 'Fucking someone is not so important that it leads to orgasm.'

Pain (n = 71)

Although physical pleasure is an important reason for some men to fuck, pain is a more common reason not to. Seventy-one men mentioned pain, hurt or discomfort, almost exclusively in the context of being receptive. The sensation ranged from mild unpleasantness to excruciating pain: 'I find passive quite painful, and I have done it with people who are quite careful.' 'Being fucked was excruciating. Have fucked in the past but never that successfully, too painful.' The pain aspect of being receptive is not constant, and various factors can influence whether it is painful or not: 'Being passive can hurt if they're not careful.' 'My present partner is far too big to do it to me.' 'It's always hurt or been uncomfortable, except when I've been drunk.' Also the pain in being receptive seems to diminish with practice (as reported by Masters and Johnson, 1979): 'I liked it only after first few times, painful at first.'

Pain, however, was not always experienced as negative: 'With being fucked I enjoy the pain of being penetrated, as I enjoy being constipated to some extent.' It is not exclusively associated with being the receptive partner: 'I find it very painful to fuck someone (if someone really wants me to I'll do it but have to like the person a lot first).' Response to the statement 'The pleasure of fucking outweighs any pain that's involved' was closely associated with whether or not the respondent had been fucked in the last year, both with casuals and regulars. Of those who agreed, 35% had been receptive with a casual partner compared with 21% who disagreed ($\chi^2 = 9.96$, df = 2, $p < 0.001$). Similarly, of those who agreed, 58% had been receptive with a regular partner, but only 37% of those who disagreed had ($\chi^2 = 15.77$, df = 2, $p < 0.001$).

Closeness (n = 40), Love (n = 25), Intimacy (n = 19) and Bonding (n = 8)

Emotional and interpersonal factors were mentioned by more men than were physical aspects. Most common among these was the closeness generated or confirmed by the act: 'Good to get close to someone.' 'A closeness is the best word.' This closeness was expressed as being both physical and emotional: 'Being attached to, being inside of, feeling a part of, possibly as close as I could ever get to somebody physically.' '. . . the closeness, a physical symbol of emotional closeness.' Fucking was represented both as a method of achieving closeness: 'Emotionally it's important, it makes you feel close to someone' and as an act that is done only with people with whom one is emotionally close: 'With a partner who I was close with it's something I'd want to do . . . it's about closeness and opening up to each other.'

Surprisingly, response to the statement 'Fucking with someone is the closest thing you can do' gave no indication of engagement in the past year in either modality, with either kind of partner. This may well be because, although fucking is a close thing to do, respondents were reacting to the superlative in the item. It is not the closest thing you can do, especially if you count non-sexual activities: 'No, it's sharing money!'

Linked to closeness was intimacy: 'It's a sign of intimacy.' 'Certainly for me it has a sense of intimacy which, truthfully, I don't get from any other form of sex.' Fucking was seen both as something that generated intimacy and was done with men with whom you were intimate: '. . . it creates an intimacy.' 'If I feel intimate towards him then I'll fuck with him.' Closeness and intimacy were also expressed in terms of bonding, oneness and togetherness: 'It bonds us together both physically and emotionally.' 'Because it involves penetration it's symbolic of the togetherness we feel at the time, an expression of the desire to be one.'

Both the closeness and intimacy that accompany fucking are often part of the love partners feel for each other. Fucking thus becomes a symbol of love: 'I call it an act of love.' 'There may be an element of showing your love for the person.' Love was also given as a reason for doing it: 'I suppose if I love that person it is important.' 'I need to love them to fuck with them.' The specialness of fucking as an expression of love makes some men want to 'save' it for the right person: 'It is the ultimate part of love. In the 40s, 50s, and 60s I spent a lot of time in saunas and I rarely fucked. It was the ultimate thing for someone special.' 'In my mind, when I was younger, I associated that [fucking] with romance, waiting for the right person, settling down, et cetera.'

From responses to the statements it would appear that love is more commonly prerequisite to fucking than a reason for doing it. That is, its absence with a casual partner is a more salient reason for not engaging than its presence with a regular partner was a reason to do it. Of those who disagreed with 'I have to love someone before I'll fuck with them', 36% had been receptive with a casual partner, whereas only 7% of those who agreed had done so ($\chi^2 = 33.92$, df = 2, $p < 0.001$). A similar pattern appears when considering insertive fucking with casuals: 47% of those disagreeing but only 9% of those agreeing had been insertive with a casual partner in the last year ($\chi^2 = 55.70$, df = 2, $p << 0.001$). Responses to the item did not vary significantly between those who had and had not engaged in fucking with a regular partner.

Trust (n = 33) and Relaxation (n = 32)

Many men mentioned trust: this took a number of forms, but mostly related to being fucked. Being able to trust the partner to stop if asked to was common: 'A bit of trust is necessary and in one night stands you're not sure how much you can trust them, to stop when you want them to.' Although trusting casual partners was a general issue, prior experience of force was given as a concrete reason not to fuck, especially with casuals, by seven men: 'It's to do with a level of trust and I need to know more than if I'd just met them 5 minutes ago. The reason is I had a couple of bad experiences in my early 20s. Me being fucked when I didn't want to be. I've been very cautious since.' Trusting the insertive partner to use condoms properly, and to check the condom periodically, also featured, and lack of trust to do this was a reason for not engaging: 'It's important to trust the partner. My ex-partner gave me trust, it could be done safely and enjoyably, I knew he'd be careful with condoms.' 'Also, having to rely on the other to keep track of the state of the condom is too much trust to place in someone else's hands and enjoy the experience.'

As with many of the above themes, trust appears both as a prerequisite to fucking: 'I need to trust them to fuck with them' and as something fucking symbolises: 'It can be a sign of mutual trust.' One of the most common reasons given for trust being prerequisite was the need to relax in order physically to achieve the act without pain, and that one needs to trust the partner in order to relax: 'In this relationship I prefer to be passive, partly because it's him, I trust him and can relax.' 'It's a question of trusting them for being fucked, I find it uncomfortable, need to be relaxed.'

Responses to the statement concerning trust were significantly associated with being fucked by a casual partner. Among those who agreed with 'I need to trust someone before I let them fuck me' only 19.3% had been fucked by a casual compared with 56.2% of those who disagreed ($\chi^2 = 41.94$, df = 2, $p << 0.001$). Response to this statement was also associated with insertive fucking with casual partners in the previous year: 28.6% who agreed had fucked a casual compared to 53.4% who disagreed; $\chi^2 = 16.81$, df = 2, $p < 0.001$). This is attributed to the fact that fucking casual partners in the last year was much more common among those who had been fucked by a casual also (67.8% versus 21.5%, $\chi^2 = 82.71$, df = 1, $p << 0.001$).

Power (n = 39), Dominance (35) and Control (n = 16)

Another understanding men either held, or recognised others as holding, was the power involved in fucking. This was usually expressed as the fucker having power over the fucked, by dominating or controlling him: 'It's partly as a demonstration of dominance over someone, you have a lot of power over someone, whether its implicit or explicit.' 'It's all about power, isn't it.' For some men the power aspect was perceived as positive, pleasurable and erotic. They liked this when doing the fucking: 'Makes you feel dominant. I like the idea of having dominance, and fucking someone gives me a sense of power' and when being fucked: 'I just like to feel powerless when being fucked, someone having power over me.' The possibility of enjoying the power from both sides was evident: 'I suppose there's more of a power difference involved than other acts which is one of the reasons I enjoy it either way round.' For others, the power was perceived negatively: 'I have never felt comfortable with being active because of the power thing behind it. Thought of the other person may not be enjoying it.' For yet others, their evaluation of the power was equivocal: 'If I analyse it deeply it's probably because I enjoy the dominance I have and the submission of the partner. I don't like that when I think about it, but I think it's true.'

Even if the respondent did not view fucking as an expression of power, many were aware of the potential the act had, and that others viewed it this way: 'It doesn't feel to me it's about power, that's been laid on by other people.' Sometimes the power relation was implicit in the language the men used. 'Dominant' and 'butch' were used synonymously with being insertive; effeminacy with being receptive: 'You can never tell from people's attitudes, you meet someone who is effeminate and they turn out to always fuck and likewise someone who is butch when you get them into bed are very effeminate sexually.' 'I'm seen as dominant so pick-ups want to be fucked.'

Men often found it difficult to articulate why being the insertive partner was being dominant, or having power. However, a few gave possible reasons: 'I enjoy the active role more than the passive, mentally I like it, dominance over someone, invading someone else.' 'I think in gay circles, like straight circles, being active is seen as something important to their masculinity.' The power aspect of fucking came to the fore for some in SM sex: 'On the odd occasion when we use bondage it's the feeling of superiority, of being master, the dominant aspect of it. It's not there when not doing bondage.' 'Now an element of bondage has come into our sex. They go together, SM, fucking and bondage.'

Holding an understanding of fucking as power often influences who fucks whom: 'There is a psychological link. If I'm going to get fucked I prefer someone older or bigger, otherwise I prefer to fuck.' 'My desire with someone younger is to be active, to do with power and experience giving.' Although the respondents almost overwhelmingly placed the power with the insertive partner, it is important to note that this is not always the case: 'Being fucked gives me a sense of dominance and power which is important to me, in the sense of a game. They're doing something under my instruction.' 'I was 18 when I met him, and it was six months before he fucked me for the first time, and that was the first time I'd ever been fucked. That was the first time I knew what I had in terms of control. Although he was the dominant one I had control because I had something that he wanted.'

Although many men made the association between fucking and power and dominance, only 30% of men agreed with the statement 'For me fucking is usually a form of domination', and only 8% agreed with it strongly. Response to the statement was significantly associated only with fucking a casual partner; 43.2% of those who agreed had done this compared with 28.2% of those who disagreed ($\chi^2 = 8.84$, df = 2, p = 0.012). This possibly reflects the belief that the power aspect of fucking was more prominent with casual than with regular partners: 'Casual sex tends to be more about power than emotion, fucking is part of power and submission . . . either wanting someone to dominate over you or dominate over someone else. With a regular, fucking is enjoyable but of reduced importance, not some power meaning, more natural, more mutually pleasurable.'

HIV (n = 126)

The way HIV relates to these men's understandings of fucking varies enormously, and the links drawn between HIV and their own behaviour are very diverse. 'It is the thing that is most associated with HIV infection, it's imbued with that significance. I couldn't do it without thinking about the association.' '[Fucking is] vital because of people being frightened out of it by HIV. It's good for me being fucked, sometimes it's what I need, no amount of mutual wanking is going to replace a good fuck. I'm making a statement "I'm not going to succumb to being frightened by HIV", a psychological statement by gay men.' 'Now though it's a very significant thing to do because of risks involved. HIV has put a completely different emphasis on fucking.' 'I'm a bit blasé about HIV, it's not something I think about all the time.'

Where a man was in his sexual career when HIV became an issue is important. For most of those who came out in the last ten years, HIV has always been an aspect of sex: 'It's a sexual act I want to do if I'm attracted to someone . . . I came out after AIDS so I've always had the same attitude.' 'I don't feel [fucking] is important for me in sex because I came out in 1983/4 when HIV was around so I never really missed it.' It was fairly common among those who had not engaged, or done it very rarely before HIV, to say HIV had put them off, otherwise they would have 'persevered': 'AIDS plays a part, if there wasn't a major risk from fucking then I'd be more tempted to work some things through about it, but it's not a major problem to me.' 'It's a form of sex that's never really appealed to me. I've tried it both ways, but didn't get particular pleasure out of it. If not for AIDS I might be willing to experiment with it.' For men who were already sexually active in the early 1980s, HIV became another consideration. Although some portrayed gay sexual life 'before AIDS' as 'the good old days': 'I had my day fifteen years ago when I could fuck people as much as I wanted, I feel sorry for young people now.' It is important to resist an image of the times pre-HIV as completely 'free and easy': 'I've always been scared of catching something, now it's AIDS, but it used to be gonorrhoea.'

How men have reacted to their knowledge of HIV (especially after it became clear that fucking was the most effective and common route of transmission between men) has been dependent on their enjoyment and understandings of fucking. The most common comment on HIV among those who enjoyed it was that it had prompted them to be more 'careful' (n = 50). This 'care' took a wide variety of forms, as people's understandings of safer sex vary, as do acceptable risks. They include: 'Before HIV I did more fucking, both ways. I've definitely reduced fucking 'cos of HIV.' 'In the recollectable past I've only fucked with friends because of HIV. If there was no HIV I'd do it more with others too.' 'HIV has made me take more precautions. I used to have lots of regulars prior to HIV. Now I'm in monogamous relationship there's no fucking with casuals.' 'Less cum through fucking than in the past because of HIV.' 'Because of HIV I try to be careful. Using condoms.' 'Part of my safe sex strategy is to have casuals in situations where fucking is not on.'

Those men who cite HIV as a major reason for them not engaging in fucking are those who did not like it irrespective of HIV: 'The overriding issue is the HIV risk involved but the whole idea of fucking doesn't appeal to me at all.' 'I have never fucked or been fucked, it is not important to me and due to AIDS I have never done or will ever do it.' Others who did not like fucking said HIV has provided an explanation to give to partners as to why they did not want to do it: 'I basically don't like it. It was fortunate that when safer sex guidelines appeared they fitted into my sexual tastes anyway.' 'I don't need to fuck with men. [HIV is a] convenient excuse not to. I like the way the spotlight has moved off fucking. It's inflated as an idea, an all-the-way moral pressure.'

These data indicate that very few men who enjoyed fucking, and got a lot out of it, have stopped doing it altogether because of HIV. Most have made their activities less risky by a variety of risk reduction strategies. The men who have stopped fucking are those who did it infrequently, and did not particularly like it.

Fucking with Regular and Casual Partners

Many quantitative studies, including Project SIGMA, consistently find fucking to be more common with regular sexual partners than with casuals (e.g., Schmidt *et al.*, 1992, McKirnan *et al.*, 1991; Sasse *et al.*, 1991, Connell and Kippax, 1990). This is reflected in the reports of these men: 'The majority of times I've fucked have been in relationships.' 'With my lover it's quite important but with casuals it's not.' 'I just don't fuck with anybody but my regular partner.'

All the preceding themes are pertinent to why fucking is more important in relationships than with casuals. Men cited emotional and interpersonal aspects: 'The actual physical side of it is not that important. It's the fact that there's a relationship there. I enjoy all sexual acts more if I feel something for the person.' '[Fucking is] more enjoyable with regulars because I know them and care for them'; temporal reasons: '[Fucking] tends to become more important the longer a relationship goes on simply because it expands the range of activities as time goes on, you get bored doing the same thing'; and HIV: 'I'd think twice about fucking with casuals because of complications due to infection.' 'I used to fuck with casuals, but don't now. Too much risk with casuals as condoms frequently break, don't know status of casuals, wouldn't believe them anyway.' However, some explained why, for them, the reverse may also be the case: 'I tend to enjoy fucking with people who are less adventurous in bed, to have more adventurous sex you need to know more about the person. If you're just picking someone up it's easier to just get into fucking, perhaps because of laziness.' 'I'm not sure why but fucking's easier with a casual partner. Somehow you just think about it less. There's something about casual sex which is more spontaneous. With a regular one thinks in terms of the relationship and what you did last time tends to inform what you do this time, whereas with casuals there's no past to draw on.' 'If you're having a more casual relationship then fucking is important to find out what it would be like with them, it's the build up to finding it's the same with them. Once you're in a relationship sex becomes less important than things like companionship.'

Many said the main reason they fucked was because their partner enjoyed it: 'I do it because my partner desires it.' 'I always think I can take it or leave it so if the other person isn't bothered then it doesn't matter; when it does it's usually because the other person wants to.' This consideration, to please the partner, is more pertinent with regular partners than with casuals. There is perceived to be more to gain in regular relationships from doing things primarily for the other person: 'If my regular partner was very keen to do it then I would, but not with casuals.' 'I hadn't really until my current partner. Very important to him. I really wanted to carry on going out with him. I decided to shift preferences to stay with him.'

Masters and Johnson interpreted their laboratory observations of fucking as involving the receptive partner providing a 'service' (Masters and Johnson, 1979), and as already mentioned, this is often how fucking is portrayed, with the receptive partner doing it for the insertive partner, with little or no pleasure for himself. This picture is not borne out by the testimonies of these men. Although a few said they were receptive for their partner: 'Being fucked is down to pleasuring and pleasing my partner.' 'It's a queen's duty'; it was far more common for them to say they were insertive, even though they do not particularly enjoy it, because their partner gains a lot from being receptive: 'My partner likes to be fucked every so often, I feel pressure on me to do it to him.' 'If I fuck someone it's usually because I'm asked.'

Collective Understandings

Men interviewed as part of Project SIGMA do not self-define their sexual otherness by intercourse, either fucking or being fucked. Nearly all of them (88%) disagreed with the statement, 'I wasn't fully gay until I'd been fucked.' Similarly, they do not define sex by fucking: 87% disagreed with 'Only fucking is real sex.' However, this activity is still subject to greater reflection than other sexual acts. For those men for whom fucking is at least sometimes important, and they are in the majority, it becomes important because it has meaning beyond physical and erotic pleasure. Even when this symbolism is resisted, its strength is evident; one respondent, while explaining his understanding, said: 'That's how I think, not particularly how I wish I thought. I wish I saw it more like other sexual acts, as physical things without meaning except pleasure.'

From item responses we can say that fucking is generally something that gay men see as a unique experience (82% agreed with 'You can't know what it's like to have been fucked unless you've done it') and that it is strongly associated with trust (73% agreed with 'I'd need to trust someone before I'd let them fuck me'). It is not seen as being a defining factor of sex nor of being gay. It is not used as a commodity to be exchanged (85% disagreed with both 'In the past, I've fucked

Table 10.1. Likes and Dislikes about Condoms

Likes	%	Dislikes	%
Protects	42.8	Loss of sensitivity	58.8
Erotic	24.0	Interrupts	56.7
Physical attributes[1]	14.8	Physical attributes[1]	36.3
Hygiene	8.9	Disposal	13.2
Improves performance	4.3	Risk of breaks	12.6
Novelty	2.5	Fiddly	11.4
Other	2.8	Uncomfortable	10.2
		Artificial barrier	8.0
		Cannot feel semen	2.8
		Other	8.0

Note: [1] Physical attributes include taste, smell and feel.

with a partner just to keep him from straying' and 'In the past, I've used fucking as a bargaining tool'). They do not see being fucked as endangering a masculine identity (82% disagreed with 'Being fucked compromises my masculinity', and 90% disagreed with 'Being fucked makes me less of a man').

Fucking and Condoms

Many people could be forgiven for thinking that 'safer sex' = 'condoms'. A large amount of energy of a number of agencies has been put into promoting condoms, especially, though not exclusively, since they have been shown to be an effective barrier against HIV transmission as well as other infections. Using condoms for anal intercourse was uncommon, though not unknown, before HIV. Most men associated them with contraception, and consequently did not view them as one of their sexual accessories. There is evidence that a large-scale uptake of condoms among gay men has occurred in the last ten years (see Weatherburn *et al.*, 1991, for a review). In this section we will look first at what respondents said they like and dislike about condoms; then at how they influence the decision to engage in anal intercourse; and, finally, at the reasons men give for not using condoms when anal intercourse does occur.

Likes and Dislike of Condoms

In wave two 325 respondents were asked what they liked and disliked about using condoms. Table 10.1 summarises their responses. The most common positive aspect of condoms was the protection they afford (42.8% of men mentioned this). The majority explicitly mentioned protection against HIV, although some said they were using condoms before HIV as protection against other infections such as syphilis and gonorrhoea, and the few who used them during vaginal sex mentioned their contraceptive value. Almost a quarter (24%) said that they found using condoms a turn-on. Men enjoyed putting them on (and taking them off) themselves and others, incorporating them into 'foreplay' and using them as a sex toy. For some men, the presence of condoms increased their sexual excitement as they were associated with fucking and anticipated pleasure. These responses validate attempts to eroticise condoms over the last ten years.

The next most common set of likes about condoms concerned their physical attributes particularly the way they felt. Although only a very few said they actually liked the smell or taste of condoms, many more said they liked the way they felt when they were wearing them. This was described as a general feeling of comfort, and of them being tight, enclosed or contained, a sensation some men found pleasurable. Other positive aspects mentioned by fewer men were general hygiene, that they improve sexual performance and their novelty value.

As can be seen from Table 10.1, there is a greater number of reasons given for disliking condoms than there are reasons for liking them. Most common were the loss of sensitivity when wearing them (58.8%), and that they interrupt the flow of the sexual session (56.7%). More than twice as many men said they disliked the physical attributes of condoms than said they liked them. These objections were mainly based in their smell and taste.

What to do with condoms once they have be used and the effort involved in getting rid of them were mentioned as a drawback by 13.2%, and a further 10% said that they were either 'fiddly' or difficult to use, or that they were uncomfortable. That condoms sometimes break is recognised by most men. This important point, and how it influences the decision to fuck, will be discussed further below. When asked what they dislike about condoms, however, only 12.6% mentioned the fact that they break. Prieur's (1990) contention that some men do not use condoms because of the symbolic barrier and distance they represent gains some support here, as 8.0% mentioned they disliked these aspects of condoms, and a further 2.8% said condoms stop the pleasurable feeling of semen being exchanged.

'I Don't Like Condoms So . . .'

The likes and dislikes of condoms that the men in the cohort reported are not dissimilar to lists reported in other studies. It is important, however, to distinguish likes and dislikes from reasons for non-use, since disliking condoms is neither a reason nor an excuse for not using them. It is also important to recognise that the decision to use a condom is not one that is taken once the decision to engage in anal intercourse has been made. Attitudes to condoms can influence the decision to fuck. For example, a man who simply finds condoms unacceptable may decide to omit anal intercourse from his repertoire. On the other hand, those who find them intensely erotic might be more inclined to fuck. We thought it crucial to ask separately about reasons for using or not using condoms in particular circumstances.

While talking about their experiences of anal intercourse at wave four fifty-nine out of 472 men mentioned condoms. The accounts they gave show that condom use emerges from a complex understanding and appreciation of the risks and benefits, pleasures and drawbacks of condom use. Some gave opinions on condoms which support the findings above, both in their positive aspects: 'I know [a condom] hasn't spoiled anything — it just provides extra insurance.' 'Condoms are a turn on, I've used them for years.' 'When I used to fuck I'd come really quickly, so for me fucking with a condom is much better' and negative ones:

'Mentally it's all about being closer to someone, which is why I don't like condoms when we use them.' 'I can't keep a hard on with a condom on.' 'Using a condom makes it take longer, it's gungy and builds the act up to an extent that makes it difficult to do other acts, if one of you is not enjoying it.' Most recognised the fallibility of condoms: 'Even with a condom there's dangers, the condom could tear or slip off.' 'Condoms are not safe, safer, but not safe, condoms split.' 'Fucking with a condom is more risky than not fucking.' 'I don't trust condoms, if women can get pregnant using condoms then certain accidents can happen.'

However, there is no simple one-to-one relationship between what men think about condoms and whether they choose to use them. Admittedly, some who do not like them, do not use them: 'I never use condoms, I don't like them. Not because I'm anti-safe sex, I just don't like them. I get a feeling inside which tells me it's alright (or not) to [fuck someone].' This response is rare, however. Many others who do not like them, do use them: 'I've always used a condom when somebody's screwing me, but I like the idea of someone coming inside of me; gives me a warm feeling. I'd prefer not to use a condom, but I do.' 'I use condoms nearly always although I miss someone coming in me, it's a nice feeling.' 'I prefer without condom but you have to be careful these days.' Others choose not to fuck, rather than use condoms. This choice was based a number of considerations including the diminished pleasure to be had from anal intercourse when a condom was used: 'I've lost the pleasure in fucking because of condoms, I've lost sensitivity and prefer to wank.' 'I don't particularly like being fucked with a condom, so in effect I've given up.' Some disliked using them: 'I dislike the process of having to use condoms and find it not worthwhile on that account' and some had concerns about them splitting: 'I don't let anyone fuck me now, there's too much risk with casuals as condoms frequently break.' 'I don't trust condoms anyhow, therefore it's a reason not to fuck.' Choosing not to fuck because of having to use a condom if you do, can be backed up by other considerations: 'When I've fucked others it's not been as nice as being sucked. Now there's even less incentive to fuck 'cos you've got to use a condom.' 'I wouldn't get fucked now, nor fuck my regular partner because I don't know my HIV status, or anyone's, and I don't want to use a condom.' 'I had a go with my lover when we first met, but we didn't get on very well, and now with the AIDS scare one just doesn't do it, even with a condom.'

Many things, then, are taken into consideration when choosing to fuck or not, and choosing to use a condom or not. Often the decision to fuck or not will be informed by attitudes towards and opinions of condoms, and condom use may be informed by understandings of fucking — among other things.

Reason for Not Using Condoms

In wave four those men who had fucked without a condom in the preceding year, either insertively or receptively, were asked why they had not used one on those occasions. The 211 (45.1%) men who had done so gave a wide variety of reasons for not using them, which are summarised in Table 10.2 (the numbers do not sum to 211 as some men gave more than one reason). The reasons given are grouped according to what kind of response the men gave. The first and largest group includes those reasons that say a condom was not necessary because of who they

Table 10.2. Reasons Given for Not Using Condoms

Reasons given (n = 211)	% (n)
Only fuck with regular partner:	33.7 (70)
Both tested negative	17.8 (37)
Monogamous since before HIV	8.7 (18)
Monogamous now	7.7 (16)
Both partners tested positive	2.4 (5)
Presumed partner was negative	10.0 (21)
Did not orgasm	3.8 (8)
Only insertive	1.4 (3)
Loss of sensitivity	7.2 (15)
Smell or taste bad	2.9 (6)
Uncomfortable/erection problems	4.7 (10)
Don't like interruption	7.2 (15)
Got carried away	14.9 (32)
Too embarrassed	2.4 (5)
Too drunk/stoned	11.0 (23)
Condoms are no guarantee anyway	1.9 (4)
No condom was available	12.0 (25)
Partner refused to use one	7.2 (15)

were fucking with. The most common reason, given by seventy (33.7%) of men, was that they only fucked with their regular partner. When asked about this in more detail, thirty-seven (17.8%) said they and their regular partner had both tested negative to HIV, eighteen (8.7%) said they had been monogamous with their partner since before HIV became an issue, and a further sixteen (7.7%) said they were currently monogamous with their partner, and that this was sufficient reason not to use a condom.

Another set of reasons why a condom was not necessary was based on how they were fucking. Only eleven men gave this kind of reason, eight (3.8%) saying because there was no orgasm during the fucking and therefore no risk of HIV transmission, the other three (1.4%) saying they were insertive only during fucking and thought they could not pick up HIV this way.

The next set of reasons may be summarised as: 'I didn't use them because I don't like them.' Forty-six men gave reasons of this kind. Fifteen (7.2%) men said that they diminished sensitivity, and a further fifteen said that they interrupted the flow of sex. A further ten (4.7%) said that condoms were uncomfortable, or that they gave them erection difficulties, and six said they did not like the smell or taste of them.

A fourth set of reasons concerns the notion of failure. They suggest that the respondent intended to use a condom, but that some intervening factor prevented, or distracted them from doing so. This was the second most common type of reason, given by sixty (28.4%) of men. Just over half of these said that they 'got carried away' with the sex, or that they did not think about condoms 'in the heat of the moment'. Many men said they had consumed alcohol or other recreational drugs before the sex, and that this was why they did not use one. Only a few men said they were too embarrassed to bring the subject up with their partner.

Interestingly, given what the men said about condoms in the preceding section, four men said they did not bother to use condoms because they were no guarantee against HIV anyway, as they frequently split or broke. The remaining two reasons, given by forty men, place responsibility for not using a condom out of the control of the respondent, by saying either that there was not a condom available (twenty-five men, 12.0%), or that their partner refused to use one (fifteen men, 7.2%).

Discussion

In this chapter we have set out at some length the wide range of understandings of and reactions to anal intercourse held by the men in the cohort. The understandings are presented by theme, rather than by person, and are not intended to be a definitive account. In particular, we are not proposing that these understandings are static. Clearly, they will change over time and vary in different contexts. Most importantly, we are not suggesting that because these men make certain responses to statements about anal intercourse they will therefore automatically engage, or be more likely to engage in, certain behaviour. For example, of two respondents who agree with the item 'Fucking is the closest thing you can do', one may be reflecting on a new relationship, within which anal intercourse is symbolic of their mutual commitment, closeness and love; the other may be a man without a current relationship but searching for someone with whom to act it out. Thus agreement with a particular item is neither necessary nor sufficient for engagement in anal intercourse.

As with other studies of primarily middle-class Anglo-American homosexual populations (Schofield, 1965a: 35; Hooker, 1965: 24–5; Westwood, 1960), this study did not find strong preferences, in terms of insertive/receptive, inserter/insertee, for the majority of men. As we showed in Chapter 9, the majority of men who fuck, do it both ways. There are, however, distinct and identifiable subjective experiences associated with each act. That the men, in general, engage in both insertive and receptive fucking (if they engage at all), allows for clarification of these differences as single individuals can introspect from their own experiences of both.

What is striking about these accounts is the relative absence of men who claim to enjoy fucking, but refrain from it because of HIV. As stated above, most of those who cite HIV as a major reason for not engaging in fucking are those who did not like the activity before they were aware of HIV. This has important consequences for studies of sexual behaviour change in response to HIV that rely on self-reported change. It is not uncommon to be given a picture of all gay men indiscriminately engaging in anal intercourse before HIV, and then being forced to stop. Those who 'persist' in doing it are construed as ignorant, fatalistic or dangerous, and there follow calls for them to be educated, modified or detained. Simplistic and gross though this representation is, it can often be heard. It is based on no reliable research, but assumption and prejudice, and it misrepresents the complexity of people's lives.

It follows, that many men who enjoy anal intercourse continue to engage in it in the time of HIV. In the next chapter we show how this is managed with a regard to safety. What the evidence does not show is that these men are irresponsible or reckless. HIV has clearly made a difference to the vast majority of gay men who have, do or want to engage in fucking. It may be worthy of note that no support is gained here for the view that anal intercourse — particularly without a condom — has become more exciting and attractive since the emergence of HIV, the 'forbidden fruit' hypothesis. Only 3% slightly agreed with 'Knowing fucking may be dangerous makes it more appealing to me.' None agreed strongly. However, many of the concerns of these men around fucking, and receptive fucking in particular, are not related to HIV, and can be assumed to have been present before we became aware of the virus. What HIV has done, in some cases, is to intensify the meanings and understandings the men hold.

Attitudes towards condoms vary greatly: some men find them a turn on, some are indifferent, some find them a turn-off. However, it is clear from the preceding review that relatively few instances of non-condom use can be explained by the fact that people do not like them. In accounting for not using them, the majority of men give rational, planned reasons for doing so. This illustrates the point that men made choices about what they are doing, based on discussion and negotiation with their partners. However, two further points need to be made about singular explanations for not using condoms.

The first is that whatever one man says about why a condom was not used when he fucked will only be half the story. The report of his partner is missing, and this gives us a biased view of what actually happens when two men decide to fuck together without a condom. In several studies, as with this one, it is not uncommon to find men who said they did not use a condom because their partner refused to use one. It is rare for the respondents themselves to admit to being the partner who refuses. This is no doubt partly a social desirability effect, but, whatever the underlying truth, it is a reason which is at best partial. To say 'I did not use a condom because my partner refused to use one' is an explanation of why a condom was not used; it is not an explanation of why unprotected fucking occurred. Answering in this way supposes that no choices were made other than by the partner, but it takes two to fuck. This is not to say that both partners are in an equal bargaining position with regard to fucking or not, and using condoms or not, but it is something that it takes two people to do.

Second, when accounting for not using condoms, it is important to bear in mind a distinction between explaining and understanding, and the limitations imposed by asking someone 'Why?' Explaining involves accounting for something that is seen as problematic, either to oneself or to other people. Understanding, on the other hand, involves seeing things from someone else's perspective, and appreciating their actions and decisions within their own frame of reference. As Wendy Stainton Rogers has pointed out:

> Most of the time people go through life experiencing it as a reasonably smoothly flowing series of events, that need to be explained or justified only when something unexpected comes along. To even ask the question 'Why did she do that?' changes things dramatically, since it implies that the action needs to be explained (i.e., was an unwarranted action, or one that broke the rules). Consequently, simply asking people to explain an action comes across as accusatory, and so invites particular kinds of response: justification, denials of blame, excuses. (Stainton Rogers, 1991: 51)

When we asked men about why they did not use condoms, they replied with exactly these kinds of responses: justifications ('I only fuck with my boyfriend', 'He was a virgin so I assumed he was negative', 'I don't think you can catch HIV from fucking someone'); denials of blame ('There wasn't a condom around', 'He just didn't want to use one') and excuses ('I was too pissed', 'I was so into him, I just got carried away'). It remains an urgent methodological issue, and one with immense practical implications, to find ways of getting behind these immediate responses to the underlying processes of negotiation, compromise and mutual understanding.

Understanding sexual behaviour means, among other things, understanding people's subjective understanding of their behaviour. HIV is not the only factor gay men consider when negotiating with a partner whether or not to fuck. It may not even be the most important; indeed, it may come quite far down their list of priorities. It is clear from the above accounts that, although structural factors play a part, interpersonal factors are of prime importance in determining sexual choice. Focusing on the interaction of partners, in the light of their individual understandings, provides a better framework for understanding their behaviour than does looking at deficiencies of knowledge, individual personality factors or temporary states such as drunkenness.

11 Casual and Regular Sexual Partnerships

'I can't even count the number of times I rolled over in bed and told some hot stranger:
You'd like my lover.'
'What about rematches?'
'Once, . . . but never again. Jon sulked for a week. I saw his point actually: once is recreation; twice is courtship. You learn these nifty little nuances when you're married.' (Maupin, 1984: 31)

As already outlined in Chapter 9, the type of relationship a man is currently engaged in (whether or not he has a regular sexual partner) is the strongest predictor of the type and frequency of sexual acts he is likely to engage in. We believe that this deceptively simple finding is a powerful means to understanding patterns of sexual behaviour, particularly anal intercourse and condom use. In this chapter we look at the kinds of organisation gay men employ for their sexual lives, and the implications for the kinds of sex they have.

Two of the most common stereotypes of gay men are that they are unable to maintain monogamous and enduring relationships, and that they are promiscuous. Gay responses to these implicit criticisms have varied: 'They're just not true, I've been with my lover 10 years and have not had sex with anyone else'; alternatively, 'Yeah I go cottaging most days and get through 40 cocks a month, what's *your* problem with that?' These two (imaginary) retorts illustrate that how many people you have sex with, and to a large extent what kind of sex you have with them, are both constrained and determined by your relationship to those people. Despite the attention which has been given to numbers of sexual partners by epidemiologists looking at the transmission of HIV, it is clear that sexual partnerships vary enormously. Fundamental to an understanding of the sexual lifestyles of gay and bisexual men in general, and of safer sexual practices in particular, is an understanding of these differing relationships and their effects on types of sexual behaviour.

To begin with, it is useful to imagine the wide variety of social contexts in which men have sex with each other, and the ways in which men can organise their sexual lifestyles. We have a huge vocabulary with which to describe sexual relations between men: lovers, boyfriends, partners, other-halves, one-offs, casuals, fuck buddies, pick-ups, trade, rent, long-time companion, etc. These various descriptions recognise that sex may take place in a wide variety of scenarios, varying from those where there is no exchange of personal information, through a whole range of interpersonal relationships, to lovers who have lived together for decades.

Before two men first have sex together, the degree of knowledge they have of each other will have an effect on the kinds of sex they have, as will their individual characteristics and expectations regarding sex. They may have known each other for varying lengths of time and in different degrees. Some pairs will have been friends for a time, others will have only met a few hours before having sex, and some may have sex almost immediately after encountering each other. In addition to exchanges of information before the first sexual encounter, where the sex takes place will have a bearing on what the men can do. As we shall see, many men have one-off sexual encounters in public places, and these locations can have an effect on what can be done sexually.

If sex occurs again, participants may have further expectations dependent on their experiences and perceptions of the first encounter. Presuming that they do recognise each other, the second session could be either by design (that is, they planned to meet again, possibly with the expectation of having sex again), or it may be by accident (they just bumped into each other). Each may have decided that there are things they would like to do that they would not have done in the first session, having thought about doing those things in the interim, or on the basis of what was most enjoyable about the first session.

As, and if, the sessions continue, the frequency of contact may have a bearing on what the men do. New ideas may develop, or one may want to do something the other does not, and over time they may introduce new sexual acts. As time goes on, trust may develop between the partners that allows them to do things they would be wary of with someone they do not know well, and the repetition of a sequence of sexual acts may prompt them to explore other possibilities. These developments are not a foregone conclusion by any means.

Bell and Weinberg (1978) found in the 1970s that whether or not a man was in a 'relationship' was the most important predictor of a number of factors in his sexual lifestyle. They designed a five-type typology of homosexual lifestyle, and despite their massive research program, they still felt it necessary to conclude: '. . . while the present study has taken a step forward in its delineation of types of homosexuals, it too fails to capture the full diversity that must be understood if society is ever fully to respect, and ever to appreciate, the way in which homosexual men and women live their lives' (p. 231). Although they conflate 'types of homosexuals' with the way people 'live their lives', they are acknowledging diversity. As they pointed out, the men in their sample enjoyed a wide range of types of relationship, but they do not pretend to account for all the ways people arrange their sexual and emotional lives.

As the above demonstrates there are a number of ways men can organise their relationships. Many previous researchers have attempted to design typologies of types of homosexuals. In Britain, Michael Schofield (1965a) subtitled his major work 'A Comparative Study of Three Types of Homosexuals'. While we recognise individual characteristics as being important, they do not determine the kinds of relationships men develop, as any relationship must take account of two people.

Rather than look at homosexual individuals, we concentrate on the types of homo sexual partnerships. This chapter will look at some of the characteristics of different kinds of sexual partnerships, and at some of the ways men organise their sexual lifestyles.

To begin with, it is necessary to clarify the distinction between 'regular' and 'casual' sexual partner that Project SIGMA used. Among regular partnerships, we also make a distinction between those that are sexually exclusive, or 'monogamous', and those that are non-exclusive, or 'open'. We then move on to consider the different characteristics of regular and casual partnerships. Finally, we consider the ways men combine regular and casual partners, and the strategies that are used to maintain regular relationships in combination with casual partners.

Regular or Casual, Monogamous or Open?

Within SIGMA a regular partner was defined as: 'a partner with whom you have had sex more than once, where the second and subsequent meetings were not accidental, and with whom you intend to have sex in the near future.' This definition includes partners who saw each other at regular intervals, be that a month or a year, who do not necessarily have an emotional or romantic attachment to each other. Nor does it confine itself to relationships that are monogamous. The definition is a statement of the relationship between two people, irrespective of their sexual activity with third parties.

The term 'casual partner' is used very simply to describe those partners who fall outside the definition of 'regular' sexual partner, and as such would not necessarily rule out partners who had sex together more than once. Because the definition of a regular partner depends on the intention to have sex again, two men could have sex a number of times, but if their meetings were accidental, they might still be counted as casual partners. Thus the term 'casual partners' covers a number of sexual scenarios which include:

> silent, or virtually silent, sex after which the participants move apart having exchanged no personal information, and would not expect to encounter each other again, in which case the sex is *anonymous and casual*;
> encounters during which a lot of information is exchanged over an evening and night, but after which the participants do not intend to encounter each other again, making the sex *casual but not anonymous*;
> sex with friends one may see often socially, and which may happen more than once, but to which no sexual commitment is made nor expectation of recurrence is attached, making the sex *occasional but still casual*.

In practice, men's sexual partnerships do not always fall neatly into the categories regular or casual. One of the more common problems was with what men usually described as an 'occasional partner'. This was where a man had an expectation and intention of the recurrence of sex with someone he had sex with before, but where no formal plans for its execution were made. The expectation usually arose because the respondent was confident that he would bump into the partner again, usually because of their shared social scene or circle, and presumed they might have sex when they met because they often had in the past. In these cases the partnership was considered regular, as the factors affecting the kind of sex they may have (e.g., location, knowledge, time scale) are more similar to those of regular partnerships than to casual ones.

Given only the categories 'regular' and 'casual', there are six different ways that men could organise their sexual partners within a given time period:

1 one regular partner and no other partners — this is what is traditionally referred to as a monogamous or closed relationship;
2a more than one regular partner and no casual partners — this could logically encompass each of three lovers who only had sex with each other, or one man who had two or more regular partners;
2b one regular partner and casuals — one regular and other casual partners;
2c more than one regular and casuals — again, this could be one of three men having sex with each other, or one man with two regulars, but also having casual partners;
3 casual partners only;
4 no sexual partners — often mistakenly termed 'celibate', a man may have had no sex by default (he didn't go looking and none came his way), design (he made a choice to be celibate), or disappointment (he went looking but didn't get any).

In this typology categories 2a, 2b and 2c may be collectively known as 'open relationships'. One major problem with this typology is what time period to take into account (Hickson, 1991). For example, if we asked people about the last week, those who might place themselves in category 3 might not have had a casual partner, and would be counted in category 4. Likewise a man who saw his regular partner/s less than once a week and had not seen him/them in the past week would move from 1 or 2 to 3 or 4. The problem is not solved, indeed it is made worse, by lengthening the time period. If we ask about the last year, a man might have had several regular partners, consecutively or simultaneously; he might have broken up with his lover last week after a long relationship; he might have had sex with no-one but his boyfriend in the last year, apart from once last month, but now they are monogamous again. Which categories do these men go in? One solution is not to use time scales to determine relationship patterns, but to ask men what *they consider* to be their *current* relationship status.

At wave four, when men were asked to describe the state of their current gay relationships, 25.1% said they were in monogamous relationships. A further 33.2% said they were in open relationships (one regular and casual accounted for 20.2%, more than one regular and casuals for 9.4%, and only 3.6% had more than one regular and no casuals). The remaining 41.6% said they had no regular partner at the moment, but none said they were celibate.

Both classification systems (self-proclaimed or based on behaviour over a given time period) have drawbacks, and there is no guarantee of congruence between them. Expectations and behaviours may differ. A couple who have an agreement of openness may be behaviourally closed, with neither of them choosing to exercise their 'right' to other partners. Conversely, within a couple who expect sexual fidelity, one or both may be having sex with third parties without their partner's knowledge.

Casual Sexual Partnerships

Here we outline the way in which casual or anonymous sex has been presumed to be synonymous with the notion of danger of HIV transmission, and then to look at the characteristics of casual sex: can we identify the type of man who has casual sex? how much casual sex do men have? where do casual partners meet, and what implications does that have for the kinds of sex they have?

Casual Sex: Anonymity and Danger?

The easy availability of sex without emotional commitment is one of the most notable features of the gay scene. Hailed by some as one of the great glories of gay culture, the availability of such sex has long been interpreted as an inability of the homosexual male to make long-term relationships (a point returned to below). Frequent casual sexual contact is often glossed as 'promiscuity', an elastic and self-reflective term with little descriptive validity. Rarely is it viewed as a positive expression of sexuality, and most apologetic commentators on homosexuality have felt obliged to denigrate it:

> The objection to promiscuity is, or ought to be, not so much the unbridled pleasure of intemperance, as the consequences such as disease, evasions, lies, thoughtlessness, self-centredness, and lack of responsibility. The fact is that even the most ardent practitioner very rarely gets much satisfaction from his promiscuity, and the feckless use of another person's body to gratify the sexual urge is a very limited and unrewarding exercise. (Schofield, 1965a: 175)

The 'promiscuous homosexual' figures prominently in the demonology of AIDS. One of the earliest authoritative epidemiological studies, the American Centers for Disease Control (CDC) case control study of 1981

> . . . identified a subset of homosexual men who were more likely to have *many anonymous sexual partners*, to have a history of a variety of sexually transmitted diseases and to engage in sexual practices that increased the risk of exposure to small amounts of blood and faeces. The most important variable was that the AIDS patients had *more male sexual partners* than the controls. (Foege, 1983: 7–17; emphases added)

Discussing this important epidemiological finding, Shilts comments: 'Patients tended to have twice the sexual contacts as the controls and to draw these contacts *from among other promiscuous men*, because they were far more likely to go to gay bathhouses for sexual recreation" (Shilts, 1987: 131–2; emphasis added). As a result of such conjecture, the American Public Health Service pledged support for local attempts to close down places '. . . where there is evidence that they facilitate high-risk behaviours, *such as anonymous sexual contacts and/or intercourse with multiple partners* or IV drug abuse (e.g. bath-houses, houses of prostitution, "shooting galleries")' (CDC, 1986: 154; emphasis added). Implicit in these accounts are the notions that anonymous sex is dangerous sex, and thus one means to curtail or even halt the epidemic is to eradicate venues that facilitate anonymous sex, and hence protect promiscuous persons from their own poor judgment. This assumption that if only gay men would conform to heterosexual norms is not only morally offensive, but is epidemiologically unsound (Patton, 1985: 135).

Nevertheless, state agencies have commonly discouraged multiple and anonymous sexual partners and extolled monogamy as a defence against HIV infection. In the United States perhaps the most important manifestation of this was the argument over the closing of the bathhouses. Shilts' discussion of the 'bathhouse controversy' (1987: 153 *et passim*) makes it clear that he regards those who defended the role of the bathhouses as being in favour of spreading the virus. Yet as gay communities came to realise the immense seriousness of the epidemic, bathhouses and other gay venues became the very places where norms of safer sex were established and maintained (Pollak, 1988; Kegebein *et al.*, 1992; Bolton *et al.*, 1992; Frutchey and Williams, 1992). As the modes of transmission of HIV became better known, attempts to popularise monogamy lost their impetus among gay audiences, and more resources were put into the promotion of safer sex. In this formulation, the number of partners was largely immaterial. Rather, avoidance of sexual techniques which involve the 'exchange of body fluids' was urged. In our terms the message was to reduce numbers of PSPs and adopt condom use for anal intercourse.

Who Has Casual Sex?

Men have casual sex for a wide variety of reasons, and there is not a 'type' of gay man who does so. Availability obviously plays a large part. From wave one, men who live in London are significantly more likely to have had a casual partner in the last year (66.3%) than those living outside the capital (58.5%; $\chi^2 = 4.187$, df $= 1$, $p < 0.05$). Within London those men having casual partners tend to be younger than those who do not ($\chi^2 = 7.985$, df $= 3$, $p < 0.05$) and say that they take safer sex less seriously ($\chi^2 = 6.549$, df $= 2$, $p < 0.05$). As the number and type of partners you have are less important to safer sex than what kind of sex you have with them, this may reflect overcaution on the part of those who are very concerned about HIV.

Outside the capital the pattern is slightly different. Casual sex seems to be associated with being sexually attracted only to men ($\chi^2 = 8.969$, df $= 1$, $p < 0.001$), engaging in sexual activity only with men ($\chi^2 = 8.097$, df $= 1$, $p < 0.001$) and being more 'out' about their sexuality ($\chi^2 = 5.021$, df $= 1$, $p < 0.05$). Paradoxically (as outness and regret occur inversely), to have more regret at being gay is also associated with having casual partners. However, it is important to stress that these characterisations by no means account for all the men having casual partners.

Numbers of Casual Sexual Partners

The number of casual sexual partners men have varies enormously. At wave one, the men in the cohort reported between 0 and 1000 casual partners in the last year.

For those who had a casual partner in the last year the median number was six, or one every eight or nine weeks, though the mean was 10.7. Fifty per cent of men had between two and fourteen casual partners, and 90% had less than twenty-three. Numbers of PSPs were far lower, with mean of 1.6 and median of none. Among the men who had casual partners 50% had no casual PSPs, reflecting the fact that anal intercourse is relatively rare in casual encounters.

The number of casual partners men have varies according to whether they have a regular partner and, if they do, whether that regular partnership is monogamous or open. Obviously, we could expect those men in monogamous relationships to have fewest, if any, casual partners, and this is the case. At wave four, those in monogamous relationships had a mean number of casual partners of 0.2 (median 0) in the preceding month. Those who did, could have started their monogamous relationship within the past month, or maybe they had a casual partner, but reaffirmed their monogamy afterwards. Among those who are not monogamous, men with an open regular relationship have on average more casual partners (mean 3.2, median 1) than those who have no regular partner (mean 2.5, median 1).

Descriptions of Where Men Meet for Casual Sex

Clubs and pubs have long been the central social venues of the gay community (Read, 1980; Bell and Weinberg, 1978; Harry and DeVall, 1978, but also Bray, 1982 and Norton, 1992, for descriptions of the molly houses of the eighteenth century, the precursors of the modern gay pub) and as such offer gay men a safe environment for social interaction and inter alia for explicit and implicit sexual negotiations. It can be assumed that the majority of successful negotiations which occur in these contexts are consummated elsewhere.

Cottages, known in North America as tearooms (see Humphreys, 1970; Delph, 1978: 64–94) and in Australia as beats (Bennett, Chapman and Bray, 1989), may be defined as any male public convenience which is known as a place where meetings may occur for sexual negotiation or contact. Not all male public conveniences are appropriate locations for sexual negotiation or exchange because of their physical location or their internal structure (see Humphreys, 1970). Also, there are fashions in the popularity of such places, partly due to periodic attempts by local authorities to stamp out homosexual activity by closure or raids by the police. Such manoeuvres would seem to be doomed to failure. Cottaging appears to have been going on since at least 1742 (Bartlett, 1988). The cottage as a social institution offers the possibility of sexual contact for a wide range of homosexually active men from those actively involved in gay politics and organisations to those outside the confines of the 'gay community' (Keogh *et al.*, 1992). Sexual negotiation is for the most part silent, and is a highly patterned and ritualized activity dependent upon and facilitated by a system of shared symbolic meanings and negotiation, guaranteeing virtual anonymity for the participants. This not only allows the married or otherwise closeted man to remain anonymous, but for others to engage in the presentation of fantasy persona (see, for example, the Orton diaries; Lahr, 1986).

Cruising grounds are usually found on lightly wooded areas such as heaths, commons and some larger parks which have become known as places where men can meet to negotiate sexual contact (see Delph, 1978). The cruising ground may be effectively divided into areas of negotiation and of sexual activity with norms of behaviour and intrusion particular to each. These areas may, however, change their boundaries or even merge as daylight fades and the possibility of intrusion diminishes.

In many parts of the world saunas and bathhouses (Delph, 1978: 135–48; Styles, 1979; Rumaker, 1978) cater explicitly for a range of sexual activity. They often include private rooms and open areas for men to engage in sex with each other and other areas for social interaction. As we have noted above, they have been the focus of much attention in the policy war around the containment of HIV infection (see Shilts, 1987; Crimp, 1989). In the UK openly gay saunas on the model of the North American bathhouses or of the saunas of continental Europe have never existed, and those few which clandestinely cater for a homosexual clientele are furtive and subject to intermittent raids by the police.

Certain beaches, or areas of beaches (Canavan, 1984), are often known locally and sometimes to men further afield as places where men meet for the purposes of sexual negotiation and sexual activity. Unlike cottages, these locales offer a relaxed and relatively clean environment relatively free from intrusion by passers-by and other beach users. These beaches often, though not always, comprise separate areas for negotiation and activity. They therefore offer fewer restrictions to intimate and prolonged sexual contact as well as a greater number of potential partners at any one time. It must be borne in mind that in northern Europe these locations are usually restricted to the summer months, and many instances of sexual activity found in our data set are beaches visited while abroad.

Obviously, men may meet on streets and public transport, in shops and cafés, in any urban centre and then move to somewhere more secluded for sex. However, this is more likely to occur in an area where there are many gay venues, or an area which has a high proportion of gay residents. Before the 1967 Homosexual Offences Act, private parties were a common form of social cohesiveness for homosexually active men and today they survive. They continue to be noted by some respondents as a source of casual partners. American ethnographic studies of male-to-male sexual contact and activity have also been made of parking lots (Ponte, 1974) and highway rest-stops (Troiden and Goode, 1975).

Popularity and Productivity of Venues

About half the men who had a casual partner in the preceding year had met at least one in a pub or club, making them the most popular places for casual sexual contacts. Twenty-seven per cent had met a casual partner in a cottage, and 26% cent had met one in a cruising ground. Despite the obstacles mentioned above, 24% of men with a casual partner in the previous year had met one or more in a sauna, admittedly sometimes abroad. Fewer had met casual partners in other locations including parties (15%), beaches (9%) and in the street (8%).

We consider the differences between these venues under two headings: popularity and productivity. Popularity refers to the proportions of our respondents who made use of the various and venues will be measured in terms of (1) the proportions using these venues; (2) the proportions meeting sexual partners; and

(3) the proportion meeting PSPs. Productivity measures the frequency or level of use made of the venues by the respondents and consists of (1) number of visits, (2) number of sexual partners and (3) number of PSPs. Both measures relate to the relative fecundity of the venues. In particular, we will be interested in the differences between the venues as sources of PSPs: of, in the broadest sense, potential 'risk partners'.

Cluster analysis identifies three separate groups of venues. The first cluster or group consists of bars and clubs; the second of cottages, cruising grounds and saunas; and the third of parties, the street and the beach. We discuss the numerical features of these groups and individual venues, and it is sufficient to note at this point that the groups do seem to have some interpretive validity.

Bars and clubs are similar venues, where socio-sexual interactions are promoted. They provide a comfortable and relaxed atmosphere, where the presumption is that everyone is gay and where an approach from a stranger is acceptable so long as certain rules are followed. Thus, while an approach may meet a rebuff, the chances of incurring hostility or abuse are minimised. Bars and clubs do not, at least in Britain, facilitate sex on the premises. Rather, men who meet each other will either repair to the home of one of them or make a date to meet sometime in the future. This has three implications for the sort of sex which eventuates from contacts made in these venues. First, the relatively long preamble to sex itself involves some communication. This does allow each of the men to assess the other, for each to get to know his prospective partner, as government HIV prevention campaigns have urged. It has been suggested that the false sense of security this knowledge gives predisposes men to have unsafe sex. Second, the communication does allow, at least in principle, the question of HIV and of safer sex to be raised; and third, it does mean that the sex will eventually take place at home, where fucking is more likely, simply because it is warm, safe and more likely to be prolonged.

Cottages, cruising grounds and saunas are, by contrast, devoted to sexual interaction in a context which is clandestine to a greater or lesser degree. An approach can only be made, therefore, once the approacher has been screened and deemed to be another cruiser. Clearly, there are degrees of difference in this group in that a gay sauna can be presumed to have a completely gay population, and it can also be presumed that a man on Hampstead Heath at 2 a.m. will be unlikely to be just taking the air. But to the extent that most saunas in Britain involve clandestine sex and many cruising grounds operate in otherwise straight areas, these venues are like cottages in the need which they impose on users to revert to a straight role when an interruption takes place. Sex often takes place in these venues, but cruisers will sometimes repair to a safer place, sometimes to the home. The type of sex which occurs in the venue itself will be such that allows quick disentanglement. Fucking is therefore relatively unlikely, unless the venue is particularly safe.

The third group consists of primarily social venues where sexual or pre-sexual contact is possible, but one must suspect that the number of streets or beaches in Britain where the density of gay men is high enough to make cruising a viable pastime must be few. To the extent that this population is mobile, however, it may be that places abroad such as the beaches of Mykonos, Sitges and Gran Canaria or the streets of Amsterdam or San Francisco feature in this category but, as we shall see, the numbers involved are relatively small.

Table 11.1. Popularity Measures for Different Venues

n = 403 Venue	% Cruising	% Meeting partners	% Meeting PSPs
Pubs	35.2	49.1	18.1
Clubs	32.0	47.1	21.1
Cruising grounds	18.4	25.8	5.5
Cottages	23.8	27.0	4.2
Saunas	12.7	23.8	3.0
Beach	2.0	8.9	1.0
Parties	7.7	15.1	3.0
Street	3.2	7.9	1.5

Popularity of Venues

In Table 11.1 the percentages of respondents (n = 403) who went cruising, met partners and met PSPs are recorded. The pattern of use in the three categories identified in the cluster analysis is clear and compelling. On each criterion, pubs and clubs have the highest proportions, followed by the cottages, cruising grounds and saunas, with the group consisting of the beach, parties and the street scoring lowest on all measures. In that last group, parties stand out as being more popular than the other two venues, though not by such a degree that we would want to reallocate it to the middle group. It should be noted that the numbers in the second column are in every case higher than those in the first. In other words, more men meet partners in the venues than typically go there cruising. This is not necessarily inconsistent. They may have made an occasional or an unusual visit and met a partner, or they may have visited some of the venues without the express purpose of cruising. It may also reflect an unwillingness to admit to cruising, which even among gay men is not always accepted and may be undertaken surreptitiously.

As sources of PSPs, clubs and pubs stand out as the most popular source from the other venues. Thirty-seven per cent of men who met partners in pubs and 45% of those who met partners in clubs met PSPs in those venues, whereas for the other venues the figures are 21% or less. Clearly, it is in this first group of venues that men meet higher numbers of risk partners.

Productivity of Venues

The second feature of the venues is their productivity: particularly the volume of partners and PSPs that each generates, as displayed in Table 11.2. In this case the pattern suggested by the cluster analysis remains intact, but one anomaly stands out, namely cottages. The first column records the mean number of individual visits made by the men who visited that venue in the past month. The ease of visiting a cottage sets it apart from the other venues in that group, with the average cottager visiting seven times a month. The second column shows the 'yield' of sexual partners per year at each venue. It is clear that the second group provides more partners than the first, with the number coming from cottages

Tablo 11.2. Productivity Moasures for Casual Partners at Different Venues

Venue	Mean number of cruises per month	Mean number of partners per year	Mean number of PSPs per year
Pubs	5.2	4.5	3.0
Clubs	3.7	4.6	2.6
Cruising grounds	3.9	5.3	2.6
Cottages	7.0	8.0	1.6
Saunas	2.8	4.9	1.8
Beach	6.4	2.4	1.0
Parties	2.5	2.4	1.2
Street	7.3	2.7	1.8

being nearly twice that from the other venues. However, this pattern is reversed and the order of the groups re-established in the third column, which records the number of PSPs met at each venue. In terms of PSPs, the street seems to belong in the second, rather than the third group.

Casual Sex: Anonymity or Danger?

We can see that there is a variety of men who have casual partners, and a variety of places where they meet them. There appears to be a definite link between where a man meets his casual partners, how many he meets, and how many of those he meets he fucks with. The majority of men meet pick-ups in clubs and pubs, although more can be met in public places such as cottages and cruising grounds. A higher proportion of those met in pubs and clubs are PSPs, compared to more public locales. Given that casual sex is more likely to be anonymous in these public locations than if the partners met in a venue where they would exchange information, it appears that anonymity and sexual risk are more likely inversely related than correlated.

Not all gay men have casual sex. About two-thirds of the group interviewed had done so in the year before interview. Nor are the numbers of casual partners and, more notably still, PSPs remarkably high. The median number of partners is six and PSPs none amongst those who had at least one casual partner. These figures do not give support to the common currency that gay men are sexually voracious, or that all casual sex is unsafe sex. As we have noted, the term 'promiscuous' is elastic in its connotation, and unhelpful in its application. Nevertheless, there are a few men who report large numbers of casual partners, and it seems that the picture of the sexually obsessive gay man relies rather on the experience of this small minority than on that of most men.

Regular Sexual Partners

As mentioned above, Project SIGMA's definition of a regular sexual partner encompasses a wide variety of relationships. Using our definition, the proportion of

Table 11.3. Numbers of Regular Male Partners for Those Who Had at Least One

Number of regular partners	Percentage with that number of regulars
1	76.2
2	9.5
3	7.5
4	2.0
5	1.6
6	0.8
7 or more	1.6

men with at least one regular male sexual partner at the time of interview varied each year, but not by a large amount. In wave one, 57% had a regular sexual partner, 64% in wave two, 65% in wave three and 60% in wave four. However, these aggregate figures conceal widespread changes at the individual level: the 60% in wave four does not include all the 57% of wave one. By wave four, the vast majority of the cohort had reported being in a regular relationship at some time in the five years.

Data on relationships that follow are drawn from wave three interviews. Of the 387 men interviewed, 252 (65.1%) had a regular sexual partner at the time of interview. We describe the different numbers of regular partners individuals had, age differences between partners, the lengths of relationships, how often the partners see each other and how often they have sex, and the characteristics of open and closed relationships.

Numbers of Regular Partners

Table 11.3 details the frequency of numbers of regular partners of the 252 men who had a regular partner. Between them, the 252 men had 382 regular partners, and the modal number of regular partners (192 men) was one. The distribution is highly skewed. The largest number of regular relationships sustained by any man was ten. This shows that the most common regular partnership arrangement is that of 'the couple'. Given the cultural commonality and prescription of this pattern, this finding is not particularly surprising. However, about a quarter had more than one regular partner. For the twenty-four men who had two regular partners, it was very uncommon for the two partners also to be sexual partners of each other. We did not in the course of interviewing encounter three men who were lovers of each other and who all cohabited. Those men who had several regular partners were often older men who had built up a network of contemporaneous regular partners, often across the country and sometimes in other countries also.

Details of the length of the relationship, the ages of the two participants, the type of sex that had occurred within the relationship and any rules or guidelines for sex outside the relationship were available for 255 of the 382 partners (88 closed and 154 open relationships), to which the rest of this section refers.

Length of Relationship

The median length of relationship was twenty-one months (mean almost four years; mode two months), the maximum being thirty-eight years. When respondents were questioned in detail about their lifetime relationship history, similar figures emerged. A few men who were interviewed no longer had sex with their regular partner, but they still lived together and considered themselves as partners and lovers. This kind of non-sexual relationship tends to have been much longer than the average.

Age Difference between Partners

The majority of work on age differences within gay relationships has concentrated on partner selection and the role of age differences in decision-making. Lee's (1988) analysis of *Advocate* personal advertisements points towards men preferring, on the whole, partners about the same age as themselves, while Harry and DeVall (1978) found that the age range 25–35 years was most desirable to all age groups, men in their early 20s preferring older partners, those 25–35 partners about the same age, and over 35s preferring younger or age-egalitarian relationships. Our own analysis of age of partner preference is similar to Harry and DeVall's (1978). When asked, 'What do you look for in a sexual partner?', 21.2% mentioned the age of the partner. Those who specified a partner older than themselves had a mean age of 25 years, those specifying someone of a similar age had a mean of 32 years, and those specifying younger partners had a mean of 43 years.

The median age difference between partners was six years (mean nine years; mode one year), the maximum difference being fifty-three years. Just over 43% of the couples' ages were within five years of each other (compared to Bell and Weinberg's (1978: 319) figure of 48%).

Frequency of Contact

Almost a quarter (22%) of men with regular partners cohabit with them. Another 40% see their partners once a week or more. Only 4% of men said they had sex with their regular partner every day, or more frequently. Most (70%) had sex at least once a week. A further 20% had sex less often than that, but very few did so less than once a month. As one might assume, there appears to be an inverse correlation between the length of time a couple have been together and the amount of sex they have: it is an old dictum, usually applied to marriage, that frequency of sexual contact declines quickly as a relationship progresses.

Open and Closed Relationships

Harry and DeVall (1978) have said that the most difficult decision facing a gay partnership is whether or not the partners are to have sex with other people. It has been found by many previous researchers that sexual exclusivity is neither an ideal nor a reality for many gay male relationships. Among the relationships at wave three, 110 men (43.7% of those in relationships) were designated at the time to be monogamous, and 142 (56.3%) were in open relationships; that is, either the respondent or his partner or both were having sex with other people, or they had an agreement that this was an acceptable possibility. Further, at least one regular sexual partner plus other partners is the most common sexual relationship configuration for all the men (36.7%).

McWhirter and Mattison's (1984) analysis of the relationships of 156 couples leads them to state that none of the relationships over five years in length was monogamous, and similar timescales have been put forward for any change to open marriage in heterosexual couples (Ramey, 1975). In this study relationships over five years in length are more likely to be open than those less than five years ($\chi^2 = 4.782$, $p < 0.05$). Of the relationships of five years or longer, 72.6% were open compared to only 57.0% of those under five years. There are, however, relationships over five years which are monogamous, but an analysis of variance of the lengths of the relationships by the type of relationship also proved significant (F-ratio = 7.938, $p < 0.05$), confirming a trend towards sexual non-exclusivity over time. This suggests that relationships usually start as monogamous and move towards openness over time. However, this is a simplification of the pattern: some start open and become exclusive over time, while others follow more complex patterns. Whether a relationship is open is primarily dependent on the needs and desires of the partners, and as these may very well change over time, so we may expect the sate of the relationship to also. This flexibility is testament to the sensitivity and openness of many gay relationships to the needs of the partners.

In terms of type of relationship the present data suggest an association between larger age differences and more open relationships. Of those couples who were contemporaries within one year, 48% were maintaining open relationships; this figure rises to 55% for those within ten years of each other and 72% for those with an age difference of over ten years ($\chi^2 = 8.230$, $p < 0.02$).

How close the partner comes to the respondent's ideal also appears to be an important factor in whether the relationship is open or not. Men were asked to describe what they would look for in an ideal relationship, and how their current partner measured up to that ideal. Of those who rated their partner as their ideal or close to it, 66% were in closed relationships, compared to 33% of those rating them neutrally, and 13% of those making mainly negative comments. However, this may just reflect flexibility and a realistic attitude to the 'ideal partner'. If the short fall is on the sexual side, men may choose to stay together, while pursuing their sexual preferences with third parties. We must not simply interpret this as meaning gay men's relationships are less satisfying than heterosexual relationships.

There are those, of course, who see in the gay refusal to privilege the sexually exclusive couple a symptom of moral degeneracy, and consider themselves vindicated by the spread of HIV. Though this stance is widespread, it is not only insulting but is not supported by our evidence. In the early years of AIDS there was much speculation that the pandemic would force gay men to abandon their 'promiscuous' lifestyles and embrace monogamy as a risk reduction strategy. For example, Blumstein and Schwartz (1983: 174) wrote: 'some of this pattern of casual sex may be changing because of a terrible disease which non-monogamous gay men run a particular risk of contracting, it is called AIDS.' Some writers thought that they had detected such a trend (McWhirter and Mattison, 1984; Hoff *et al.*, 1992) For example, McWhirter and Mattison (1984: 291) claimed: 'we

Table 11.4. Summary of Previous Studies' Proportions of Closed relationships

Year	Author	Criterion for closed relationship	Percentage
1973	Saghir and Robins	No sex with others for length of relationship	25
1978	Harry and DeVall	No sex with others in last year	25
1978	Bell and Weinberg	Composite measure	36
1980	Mendola	Considered themselves closed	37
1981	Peplau	No sex with others in last six months	46
1981	Peplau and Cochran	No sex with others for length of relationship	30
1983	Blumstein and Schwartz	No sex with others for length of relationship	18
1985	Blasband and Peplau	No sex with others for length of relationship	10
1985	Blasband and Peplau	Considered themselves closed	48

believe there is a trend towards more sexual exclusivity in the future amongst gay men. Currently it is being propelled by fear of AIDS and more and more individuals are expressing the desire for sexual exclusivity with one other man.'

As Table 11.4 illustrates, measuring changes in the proportions of closed to open relationships is difficult since researchers have used different classification systems. Assessing the impact of HIV on gay men's relationships in the UK is made more difficult as few large-scale research studies were made prior to HIV. What evidence exists is anecdotal or from biased samples (Schofield, 1965). The studies referred to in Table 11.4 took place in the United States, with varying sampling procedures, and it is problematic to make cross-Atlantic comparisons given the cultural differences, time differences and the disparate social organisation of gay men in them. These points are to be borne in mind when making any assessment of continuity or change, similarities or differences.

In the next section we explore some of the alternative strategies to sexual exclusivity men have developed in response to HIV. Although it is not possible to say whether or not the proportion of closed relationships has increased with the advent of HIV among these men (since our research began five years into the epidemic), it is clear that sexually exclusive relationships are not the preference of the majority.

Some Real Lives

As a supplement to the quantitative data on open and closed relationships, Project SIGMA carried out a large number of tape-recorded open-ended interviews with both partners in a relationship. The two partners were interviewed separately but simultaneously, in order to minimise collusion. The following is a selection from those interviews to illustrate the diversity of gay relationships, and to add a more realistic feel to these data.

A Monogamous Couple. Geoff and Rufus are both in their early 30s and have been together just over two years. They met through mutual friends and live on separate sides of a large conurbation, seeing each other a few times a week. Neither has had sex with anyone else since they met and started having sex with each other. They discussed sexual exclusivity early in their relationship. Geoff tells how that came about:

> Well, because when we were talking about feeling secure and feeling safe, one thing that came out that was very important, was that we wanted to have a monogamous relationship. I think Rufus, in addition, wanted to have a monogamous relationship because he's frightened of HIV. But I don't think that HIV's got a lot to do with having a monogamous relationship because as I suspect you know from your survey, most people that are not monogamous probably would have safe sex with their casual partners. Certainly if I was going to have another partner, I wouldn't be having unsafe sex with them anyway. So I don't think the HIV issue is an issue for me about why I'm monogamous. I'm just monogamous anyway, cause I find it hard to relate to more than one person at once.

Rufus remembers the topic coming up slightly differently, and takes up the issue of trust:

> I think the issue came up when he was explaining previous boyfriends. I think at the same time he was asking about my boyfriends as well. And he said since his ex-boyfriend he hadn't been sleeping with anybody else and he hasn't found the right person. He's not one for having casual one night stands. So that's, just the way it fits in with his whole character now. I didn't have any reservations at all. I'm not sure how I'd have felt at the time if he'd had. I don't know, the situation didn't crop up so we didn't need to address the problem. I didn't have any reservations that he was sleeping with anybody else. I think having by then [after a few weeks] got to know him, obviously not reasonably well by that time but I think you get a feeling and you can judge a person. And I didn't have any feelings that he was sleeping with anybody else and I believed him. I know now that he's a really honest person so when he said he wasn't and I believed him. I've got no reason to doubt him.

When asked if he would consider having sex with someone else should he be apart from Rufus for a time, Geoff thought he would not: 'No. I've got videos that I can watch and there's all sorts of ways of having sex with yourself. I often like to use different sort of underwear and things like that. And sort of maybe look at myself in the mirror and watch videos and fantasise about different things. There're all sorts of different things. And I can use different lubricants.' The decision not to have sex with other people was not a one-off decision, but part of an ongoing negotiation in their relationship. Geoff again:

> In fact it comes up quite a lot, about jealousy, and we have ongoing discussions about that because in fact he often looks at other men but he doesn't do anything about it. I get quite jealous about him looking, you know particularly if he's with me. If I wasn't there I wouldn't know, wouldn't bother, but I actually walk along the road with him and he's

> looking at someone and I feel quite a bit jealous. I look at other men sometimes, but I'm more subtle about it.

Rufus also recognises that being monogamous is an ongoing decision, and explains why he makes that decision:

> Yeah. It's actually a positive choice. In any relationship I'm more likely, not more likely than Geoffrey, but I'm more likely to be monogamous than not. And knowing Geoffrey a lot longer, I don't think I would have been tempted to dabble outside a relationship anyway. But certainly not now with Geoffrey cause I think I'd feel I'd upset him. And if he was upset then it would upset me. Also I don't think it would be of great sexual gratification for me. Because I know it could only be one night stands or casual partners. And I don't think it would mean anything to me unless I was emotionally involved with someone. And I couldn't get emotionally involved with someone whilst having a relationship with Geoffrey. I think even if I had a regular boyfriend on the side, I think I'd find it very difficult to relate to two men closely emotionally.

Both partners feel they benefit from being monogamous. Rufus explained the benefits for him:

> The security, knowing he's there, knowing I care for somebody. I think that give me a lot of support and warmth for me personally. And we often talked about it, it's nice not having to go out to the pubs and sort of stand around in smoky pubs feeling quite distorted, distraught as you walk away in the evening, yet again, you've got nobody to go home with. So yeah, I mean that always has a great benefit. Not having to do that. Which in some ways, 'cause some of our friends, one of them who's still single, goes up there regularly and I don't see him so much because of it. Because that was our meeting place as friends, so I don't see him as much, which is the only one regret I would have about it.

An Open Couple who are Behaviourally Monogamous. George, now his mid-20s, and Ken, who is ten years older, met six years ago at a social group, and had a six month platonic friendship before becoming sexual partners. They have shared a flat in a medium sized city since shortly after becoming partners. When they first started their sexual relationship, Ken remembers that they discussed relationships:

> We talked that first night and stayed up very late, we talked about relationships a lot and about what type of relationships we've had and what type of relationships we wanted. I can't really remember if it was the first night. I mean maybe not right at the beginning but very soon afterwards we did start talking about the reality of us having a relationship and that if we wanted to put some effort into this and spend a lot of time together. The reality now though is that eventually we are going to seek other sexual partners. But it's always been open to that. It was never 'we've got to be monogamous for the first year and then we can start'. It's always been an option.

Although always an option, the subject did not seriously come up until George and Ken were having problems in their sex life, four years into their relationship. George explained what happened then:

> I think how it came up was we were talking about the sex and what I wanted to do that he didn't, and he quite flippantly said 'well why don't you go off with someone else?' and I think I probably quite flippantly answered back 'well, maybe I will'. Then there was a great deal of negotiation about and suddenly instead of quite flippantly it was taken quite seriously and there was all sort of negotiation about sleeping with other people.

Between them they decided guidelines to allow them to have sex with other people without disrupting their relationship. According to Ken:

> It's not been as strong as 'you can do this but you can't do that'. It's more like 'this is what I would quite like'. 'This is how I would see it working'. 'what do you think'? The rules, I think, have developed over the years rather than being as an initial thing because initially we weren't sure what our commitment was. But now the rules are that, first and foremost, we are lovers with each other, or partners, and if we have sex with other people they are not to be every night. The aim is that they don't develop into partnerships. Like my main partnership in my life is with George and I will have flings or lovers but that's as far as it goes.

George elaborated on their negotiation: 'We decided that yes, we could if we wanted to. That so long as we told one another straight away so we didn't find out via another person.'

In practice, though, once they had allowed the other to have sex with other people, they found the strains on the sexual side of their relationships diminished, and since negotiating an open relationship two years ago, neither has taken the opportunity. When asked why he had not actually had sex with anyone else, George replied:

> I don't know. I don't think it's because I'm very content within the relationship. *I am* very content with the relationship, but I don't think it's for that reason. I think even though it's been talked through and we've agreed on this and we've agreed on that, I just think that when it happens all hell will break loose. I think he's quite jealous, and I think I'm quite jealous as well. It's just that I thought that if I'm going to do it it's going to be someone as opposed to just anyone for the sake of it. It's going to be someone I really like, not just taking half measures. If I see someone I really fancy then I think 'well fine' and it's reciprocated then I'll think 'fine' and I will. But I haven't up till now.

Ken gives a different explanation as to why he has not had sex with anyone else so far: 'We haven't actually done it. This is all theory. Actually for me, sexually, it's very few and far between men that I fancy enough to want to sleep with.

Basically because I think I'm lazy about getting it together to chat someone up or cruise or whatever.'

A Regular But Infrequent Open Relationship. Peter and Martin met in a gay pub two years ago, and spent a night having casual sex, which they both enjoyed a lot. Since then they have met every month or two, primarily for very satisfying sex of a type that they do not have with other people. Martin is married, and lives in another city with his wife, who knows about this relationship. They are both in their 40s, and are both very happy with their arrangement; neither wants any changes in the arrangement. Peter explained: 'As far as Martin and I are concerned, I think as we enjoy meeting each other and having sex with each other. He's married, so the idea of sexual fidelity with him has just never come up because the situation means that we couldn't possibly have that anyway, even if we wanted it. But I don't want that.' Peter does not have any other regular sexual partners, but enjoys casual sex with other men: 'I think it is something that was implicit from the very beginning. Neither of us ever set out to take this as a one to one relationship. In fact I've always gone out of my way to make sure that he knows that I don't see it as that. As far as I'm concerned I'm a free agent and do what the hell I like. And Martin's wishes on that just don't come into it.' This is a situation Martin is entirely comfortable with:

> It doesn't bother me at all. I'm not really emotionally involved, but I mean if I never saw him again, it would really upset me. But I wouldn't say I was in love with him. It's a very sexual relationship. We've both been through long drawn out emotional relationships. We've had enough, yes. In fact we've said that before. I think one or two of his casual relationships have been a bit clingy, and all of a sudden he's found it a bit tiresome. And you know, been there, done that. I don't really want that just at the moment, thank you.

Martin claims no curiosity about Peter's sexual life when they are apart: 'It's not relevant to our relationship. And like I don't ask questions about his other partners, if he talks about them he talks about them, if he doesn't I don't bother to ask questions. I've never asked him about his previous boyfriend. I never even thought about it. It's not relevant. Maybe because it's not, as I said before a romantic relationship.'

This arrangement was not discussed, but assumed from the start. However, they both find the sex they have together 'special'. Peter explained:

> As far as I'm concerned Martin is the person I have found who comes closest to most of my sexual fantasies. And I've never really thought about finding somebody who would fulfil those fantasies. I just thought they were going to be fantasies, which means we've actually been able to explore an S&M relationship, I guess. . . . Martin and I have a very different sexual relationship than I have with anyone else. Because I think to enjoy that sort of sex, it involves a great deal of trust, and an understanding of what both partners want which we have developed and because that's happened I really haven't felt a need to particularly explore that with other people necessarily. So that makes my relationship with Martin different.

Martin agreed:

> It's very rare to find somebody who you're sort of sexually compatible with and that you're on the same wavelength. Other people seem to wrap sex up in all sorts of other guises you know. They don't seem to enjoy it so much. I mean it can be better, it is better, you'll put up with a lot more with somebody you're really romantically involved with, even if the sex is lousy, if you're really fond of that person you will ignore that. But for Peter and I sex is sort of, it's really really good. It's unusually good. If I moved it wouldn't make any difference unless I moved to the other end of the country or abroad. But if I stay in this end of England, he's not that far away.

Peter thinks the ease of their relationship has been important to its success: 'Why he's turned out to be my most regular partner? I suppose the answer is that he doesn't put any pressure on me. That's the reason that most of my other relationships gradually folded.' Martin feels the organisation of their relationship makes things different than for a 'regular' couple. He commented on the way their relationship has developed:

> I think I was always a bit nervous because when you don't have that sort of build up of a relationship, maybe when you first start the relationship you see each other at least every other day or every weekend or something. Because it was never a romantic relationship we didn't see each other that often. So initially when I was coming here, not exactly nervous, but I was hyped up sexually and I was a bit hesitant as to what we were going to do this time. And gradually that nervousness or whatever it was has disappeared altogether. I think its trust really when you come down to it. I suppose I trust him more than I did at the beginning. You just learn more about somebody and the times we spent a few weekends together, we seem to get on quite well. On a certain level, well different level. I mean he comes from a totally different world than me, but we've managed to find a sort of level we can communicate on. Not just sex though.

An Open Couple Who Cohabit. Harold and Kit are both in their early 30s, and since meeting through work have been partners for three years. They share a house in the suburbs of a large city. Both of them have other sexual partners, sometimes separately, sometimes together. This has been the case since the beginning of their relationship when they both agreed on an open relationship, as both had similar wishes and attitudes. Kit explained: 'Neither one of us wanted to be "tied down" in that sense and, besides that, neither one of us believes in monogamy at all. It doesn't seem an option. To me, monogamous relationships are not an ideal so I don't ever expect monogamy from anyone and if anyone expects it from me then I'm not likely to get involved with them.' Harold holds similar views: '. . . when we realised that things were getting serious, or seemed to be, we laid our cards on the table and I said "This is what I want, this is what I expect, this is what happened before and it's not going to happen again" and he did the same thing. And for some strange reason it all fitted and we basically wanted the same thing.' They started only having sex with other people at the same time (mainly threesomes), but this changed: 'Initially, we decided we were going to work as a unit, and basically we still do, but the relationship has changed, and people change, and you've got to allow for that.'

As their relationship developed, and they started having sex with other people independently, Kit and Harold set some guidelines as to what they could do, but this was flexible. Kit explains:

> As it comes to rules, there are rules, but they are very flexible and we talk about things practically on a day to day basis and review the situation constantly. It sounds like it's easy to change the rules when you want, but it's not quite like that but it's just that, as we are people, our situations change, our responses change and a relationship should reflect that. The only rules I can think of are honesty is important, the one thing that would really annoy me would be if Harold did something and didn't tell me or told me something that wasn't so. That's the only strict rule. The other thing is that, we have to talk to each other about what is happening and get the other's opinion for example.'

Communication was seen by both partners as essential to their relationship, and the way it worked. According to Harold: 'The more we got to know each other, the more we began to discuss things which still exists now. I think the reason our relationship is so successful is because there is constant communication. Whenever there is a communication break-down, we get into trouble.' While sexual exclusivity was not a requirement of their relationship, this was not because of disregard for each other. Both saw honesty as being very important. Harold echoed some of Kit's remarks when he said: 'The only thing which would bother me would be if he lied to me. And that's not just in a sexual sense, that's in every sense. That's the one thing that upsets me. Other than that, things don't bother me.'

Open Relationships: Maintaining Specialness and Safety

As illustrated above, establishing and maintaining an open relationship requires communication and negotiation. Among couples who chose these relationships, past researchers have found a number of regulatory mechanisms. These mechanisms take the form of rules and guidelines, either explicitly negotiated between the partners or implicitly understood by them. Such rules have been found between heterosexual couples (for example, Buunk, 1980) as well as homosexual couples (for example, Blumstein and Schwartz, 1983; McWhirter and Mattison, 1984; Hickson *et al.*, 1992).

These rules have both manifest and functional components. A manifest component is about, for example, whom sex is allowed with; where it may take place; what kinds of sex are permitted; where the other partner is at the time; what is said between the partners about the sex; or the number of times sex is allowed with the same third party. A functional component can be thought of as the effects the rules facilitate; for example, there are those rules that are concerned with maintaining the primacy of the relationship, which assert it as separate and different from other sexual encounters. Another example are rules which function on a day-to-day basis to avoid confrontation and irritation (akin to agreeing to put the toothpaste top back on).

There need be no direct correspondence between the manifest content of rules and their functions. Indeed, two contradictory rules, for example, to tell the partner when extrarelational sex has taken place and not to talk about sex with third parties, may be used for the same purpose, that is, to minimise jealousy. Furthermore, a manifest rule may function, possibly unintentionally, in more than one way. For example, a rule about engaging in anal intercourse only with the primary partner is a rule that makes sex safer in terms of infections, for both partners, but it may also function in keeping the relationship special (Prieur, 1990).

Even if a couple reject a closed relationship, there can be problems that occur if either or both of the partners are having sex with other people. These can include:

> fears about the strength of the relationship;
> concerns about the physical safety of the partner when they are with others;
> problems about disruption to friendship networks should they be having sex with people known to both of them;
> anxiety about HIV.

A common way for couples to cope with these problems is to agree rules or guidelines to follow when having sex with other people. Rules tend to be tailored to couples' particular needs and concerns, and vary greatly. Many, if not most, are concerned primarily with maintaining the 'special' nature of the primary relationship, while allowing the potential for casual contact. Given that this pattern of accommodation was prevalent before the 1980s, it is plausible to assume that the need for safer sex was grafted onto this set of existing rules. In wave three those respondents with at least one regular sexual partner were asked: 'Do you currently have any rules, guidelines or understandings about sex outside your relationship?' Considering the eighty-eight relationships that were closed, the majority said that there were no rules or guidelines as they did not have sex with other people. However, some reported discussions that anticipate the rules of the open couples:

> We have an understood rule not to have other partners. My partner was away for four months and it was understood that he might, and I might, have other partners then, but neither of us did.

> We had threesomes before 1986, but not since then. If either of us had sex with someone else in the future it would have to be a threesome. We understood that from the beginning.

These rules are anticipatory. Neither partner expects to have sex with other people in the future, but they acknowledge the possibility. What these men highlight is that their monogamy is not merely a restrictive rule but an active choice.

Some understandings are explicit that HIV is an issue to be considered if outside sex does take place: 'We agreed that if we strayed there would be no fucking or cumming in anyone, or vice versa.' 'If he does it must be safe. . . .' The most common agreement within a closed relationship was that if extrarelational sex did occur, the partner would be told about it: 'If he does . . . he must tell me.' 'If we had another partner we'd tell each other afterwards.' These men recognise the possibility of sex with someone else. In principle, this minimises the emotional disturbance should one of them have sex with another, while also developing strategies that minimise the risk of HIV infection.

Of the 154 *relationships* that were open, 72.7% (n = 112) had some agreement between the partners as to the nature of sex with third parties. One feature of these rules and guidelines is their diversity. Some of the rules reverse rules within other relationships. Consider the following pairs:

> My partner can bonk women but not men.
> Generally, not to have sex with women as it's found more threatening.
>
> If we pick someone up it must always be in our flat and never theirs. . . .
> Never at our home. . . .
>
> We should tell each other.
> Not to talk about it.

The following analysis of the rules concentrates on their manifest rather than functional content. As mentioned previously, the same rule may function in two opposing ways. Conversely, two rules that appear contradictory may facilitate the same outcome.

Rules about Information and Honesty

The first type of rule is about information and honesty. Twenty-eight open relationships involved such an understanding. Anticipated by the pre-emptive rule within the closed relationship mentioned earlier, these agreements often take the form of telling the partner when sex has occurred: '. . . being totally honest.' 'I do not like to be deceived and we don't pretend that nothing has happened.' '. . . we're supposed to tell the truth.' In this last quote we see a recognition of the fragility of the rules. Some rules demand that the partner knows before the sex occurs: 'The partner must know and give permission. . . .' 'We have to tell each other first or immediately afterwards.' Some rules concerning information are more pragmatic and aim at reducing worry: 'We must tell each other what's happening, e.g., if we stay out all night.' 'If I go out I must tell him where I am so he doesn't worry.' Yet others suggest a sharing of the sexual experience by recounting the session in some detail: 'Each tells the other exactly what happened.' '. . . if I take someone back for sex I must give my partner an account in the morning.'

Rules about Regularity and Emotional Distance

While rules about information and honesty can serve different functions, the following set concentrates on maintaining the primacy of the partnership. They were present in twenty relationships. These rules emphasise that other sexual relationships are different; that they are 'only sex'. Often they prohibit seeing another partner more than a set number of times, or curtail the regularity of seeing them: 'Casuals are OK, one offs. We must not go back to someone twice; that would be a relationship.' 'We're not allowed to have partners we see more than once.' 'We can go with others as long as it's not more than two or three times.' Another rule that kept extrarelational sex 'just sex' was: 'No sleeping with anyone else.' Others couched this rule in more explicit terms, concentrating on both partners' feelings for and emotional attachment to each other: 'That outside relationships are not threatening.' 'We think it's important for us to have sex with other people, that way our needs are met. Our relationship is central though, our prime loyalty. If someone gets too close it will be discussed. It doesn't happen for me so it's no problem, but for him it does because he forms deeper relationships.' 'The unwritten rule is no emotional involvement.'

Rules about Discretion and Politeness

Rules about regularity and emotional distance are aimed at sustaining the relationship as primary. They concern themselves with making sure nothing occurs that could damage the stability of the relationship. A third group of rules aims at avoiding irritation and hurt feelings: 'We mustn't offend each other's sensibilities in the execution of infidelities.' 'Don't bring people back to the house when the other is there. It's an implicit rule out of politeness.'

In some cases a mode of operation has developed that bridges the underlying principles of keeping the relationship primary and facilitating discretion: 'We wouldn't walk off with someone in front of each other.' 'If we go out together we go home together.' The problem of not being seen to choose someone else over the partner can be achieved more simply: 'We don't go cruising together,' or by restricting extrarelational sex to times when sex between the partners is not possible, for example: 'We wouldn't have sex with people in Britain, but we're allowed casuals in Amsterdam or Thailand.' '. . . only away from our own town.' These last two examples, while involved with issues of discretion, also safeguard the primacy of the partnership. Eighteen relationships had negotiated rules about discretion and politeness.

Rules about Threesomes

Seven couples had found that they could both have sex with other people, without having to think about their partner having sex with someone else instead of them, by doing it at the same time: 'We only sleep with other people if it's a threesome. This was a joint decision when we discussed the possibilities of do's and don'ts.' 'No outside partners unless it's in a threesome. We decided that this was OK and not threatening.' This rule can be part of a larger objective that satisfies both partners: 'The rules are; one, we work as a team; two, we have to both pick someone up or go as a threesome; three, no fucking with others without a condom. . . .'

Rules about Safer Sex

By far the most common type of rule among these couples concerned safer sex: 43% of open relationships had some kind of agreement as to what kind of sex partners could have outside that relationship, usually based on safer sex guidelines. These rules take a variety of forms and illustrate the different ways people construe 'safer sex'. They included acts prohibited: 'He doesn't like me to fuck or have someone come in my mouth.' 'Always safe sex, no fucking even with condoms.' 'Sexually, no fucking at all' and acts proscribed: 'It has to be incredibly safe, mutual wanking only, as we don't have safe sex ourselves.'

Where there was no restriction on anal intercourse with others per se, many men mentioned an agreement about condom use with outside partners: 'It must always be safer sex, I'm allowed to fuck and be fucked with condoms.' 'No fucking with others without a condom and obey all safer sex rules.' 'It must all be safe; always with a condom and no taking of semen.' Some of these rules were occasionally elaborated on, the man going on to say that he did not have safer sex with his partner: 'We screw each other but have safer sex with other people. This has been the case since we met. We both knew the realities of the risks.'

Rules about anal intercourse did not always develop due to safer sex. The symbolic importance of this act in a regular relationship, as an act of love and/or trust, can result in partners not wishing to do this act with others, a point discussed in the last chapter: 'We've both talked about sex with other people. My partner wouldn't fuck because of his love for me; having a wank is OK.'

12 Conclusions and Implications

HIV prevention programs are bedeviled by their own success. There is no praise for seroconversions that do not happen, for lives saved or communities protected. The reward for success is, rather, to be accused of scare-mongering, of demanding special treatment, of foisting a gay liberationist agenda in the guise of health promotion. As the high media profile of HIV lowers, as ring-fencing of funds is ended and as the contract culture of the new National Health Service allows the prejudice of managers to influence and perhaps override clinical judgments, we can expect to see many of the successes of the 1980s debilitated or destroyed. Resisting and challenging these changes is, ultimately, a question of political will. As we have suggested in Chapter 2, there is space in the chronicle of the 1980s for a little pride, some satisfaction, a few plaudits for the successes, insubstantial though they may sometimes seem in the greater devastation. The work of Project SIGMA combines retrospect and prospect. On the one hand, we are able to show the success and the failures of HIV prevention policies and initiatives among gay and bisexual men. On the other, we seek to point to new directions, fresh challenges, emergent problems. We will not be alone in this, nor do we claim any greater right to dictate the future directions of policy than any other group. This final chapter we devote to a consideration of the findings we have outlined above and a series of suggestions for the future.

The Good News

There is good news in our study, which it is sometimes easy to disregard, so preoccupied are we with the identification of tasks still undone, challenges yet unfulfilled. There follow some of these items.

Knowledge of HIV, safer sex and associated matters is high

Almost no-one in the cohort was dangerously misguided about these important matters. The task cannot, however, simply be regarded as complete. There will always be new recruits to the ranks of the sexually active and to the gay community. They cannot, given the dearth of information about homosexual practice in general and safer sex in particular, be assumed to have such knowledge, and there will be, for the foreseeable future, a role for continuing campaigns conveying basic information.

But knowledge is not static. As we have shown elsewhere (Hunt *et al.*, 1991b, 1993), the growing scientific conviction that oral sex is relatively safe from the point of view of HIV transmission is reflected by an increasing engagement in the cohort over the period of the project. Such changes in expert knowledge need to be shared. This is best done, as in the past, by responsible and reasoned reporting in the gay press.

Similarly, as basic information becomes well integrated into the daily lives of gay and bisexual men, so is there scope for more detailed information to be disseminated and made widely available. Thus, for example, as condom use becomes more usual, so information about different types, the suitability of different lubricants and safe use needs continually to be made available. There remains a place, therefore, for basic and more sophisticated information campaigns.

Safer sex is remarkably widespread

It is easy to forget that until a decade ago safer sex was unheard of, so the universal knowledge and the widespread practice of safer behaviour is the more remarkable. It is important to avoid complacency on this, however. The short time it has taken to establish safer sex points also to its potential fragility. In the immediate future a balance needs to be struck which acknowledges the continuing need for safer sex and at the same time avoids overstatement or generating needless panic. In the early 1980s the gay press was remarkably successful in making news about HIV and safer sex widely available without screaming headlines. In the future a similar program of insistent but low key information and encouragement is needed, built into the fabric of gay culture, not standing monolithic and alien within it. As we write, there is a noticeable increase in the number and range of gay publications available. While it is not possible to say whether this will continue or whether any or all of these will become established, we are heartened by the way in which issues of safer sex are treated within these increasingly diverse pages: with humour, sophistication and responsibility.

HIV and safer sex have become normalised

This trend towards incorporating safer sex within existing and other concerns, treating it as inescapable but as only one facet of gay experience, is an important one. Many gay men have devoted our professional lives to HIV and its effects. Sometimes it is easy to forget that for many other men HIV is less central to their existence, less important in their views of the world. There is a tendency among some activists to see in this a denial of the fact of HIV, but this is fundamentally misguided. In our view the task of health promotion should be to encourage normalisation, while avoiding complacency — a simple prescription, but a difficult enterprise.

Safer sex practice is becoming more sophisticated

As we have shown in Chapters 10 and 11, the practice of safer sex has moved from the tactical to the strategic. In the early days of the epidemic particular practices were simply avoided by many if not most men. As time passed, however, the practice of safer sex became set within a strategic regard, a development of what the Australians have called 'negotiated safety' (Kippax *et al.*, 1992). This embedding of safer sex practice within relationship structures and understandings has led some commentators to conclude that unsafe sex is on the increase. This is, as we have pointed out previously, fundamentally mistaken. What we are seeing, we believe, is the development of risk minimisation strategies in the place of risk elimination. We have been critical in the past of researchers who have sought to condemn this — to our minds — wholly sensible strategy as 'relapse'. Here we repeat our conviction that the task of research is to track these changes. The task of health promotion is to enable them to ensure that they are as safe as possible.

The Not So Good News

As we have indicated in earlier chapters, our cohort overrepresents the middle-aged, middle-class, educated white gay man in urban centres of the UK. Any evaluation of our findings must attend to the possibility that the findings do not automatically apply to other groups. It may be that we have here interviewed the most responsible, the most enlightened, the least unsafe, but this must remain at best a presumption, at worst a misguided prejudice, for it is easy to overstate the problem and in so doing run the risk of becoming paternalistic and dismissive. While it is a possibility that working-class men or black men (who, while certainly underrepresented, are not absent from the cohort) will think and act differently from the middle-class white men in our cohort, it is not necessarily the case. Indeed, to the extent that the latter group report sexual activities with men from these other groups, there is reason to believe that they will, in fact, think and behave in quite similar ways.

Moreover, we recognise in this caveat — which we have often heard put forward as a criticism — a species of chauvinism and one which is all too prevalent in the research community. The assumption behind this criticism is often that the middle-class gay men in our sample, because we have shown them to be on the whole responsible and sensible, are the good guys and that the bad guys, those who continue to behave irresponsibly, are those about whom there is little or no research evidence: the working class, the black men, young men (but see Davies *et al.*, 1992) and those in rural areas. This presumption does not, however, stand up to scrutiny. By whatever terrible historical accident, the urban, white gay communities of North America and northern Europe have been and continue to be disproportionately affected by HIV. It does not help in the search for a realistic appreciation of individual and communal risk to point the finger at groups marginalised not only by their sexuality but also from the established gay culture.

Second, we must recognise within our cohort continuing trends of behaviour that cause some concern. We have repeatedly pointed to the increase of unprotected anal intercourse within regular relationships, along with our conviction that this is on the whole a healthy and reasonable trend. It remains the case, however, that the simple fact that a relationship is regular — in our terms — or expected by the participants to be permanent is not in itself sufficient reason for unsafe sex. In our opinion more attention needs to be focused on the processes of decision-making in these circumstances and the criteria which need to be addressed when this momentous decision is made.

Although we have spent a great deal of time on the emergence of unsafe behaviour within the relationship, it remains the case that there are still incidents of unsafe behaviour with casual partners. While it would be wrong to condemn absolutely each and every incident of unprotected anal intercourse with a casual partner, it remains a real problem. We have indicated throughout this book our conviction that the search for the individual who has unsafe sex through deficiencies of his intellect, attitude or will is misguided for theoretical reasons and unsubstantiated by empirical evidence. We believe, therefore, that future work should concentrate on the circumstances, the interaction which produce unsafe behaviour. While it might seem inappropriate to call for more research after seven years of work, costing large amounts of money, it remains the case that the process of negotiation is poorly understood.

It may be that the key to this conundrum is the recognition that HIV remains, as we have indicated in Chapter 3, a problem of other people. So long as my partner is 'like me', or at least does not conform to my stereotype of the sort of person who will be HIV positive, then unsafe sex becomes more likely. It is, however, difficult to disentangle rational risk minimisation from recklessness. The final failure is to incorporate those of us who are HIV positive within the discussion of safer sex. Implicit in many discussions is the assumption that the audience is HIV negative and the task is 'our' protection.

The Agenda

The conclusions to be drawn from our research indicate that a wide range of tasks remains important and of immediate concern. These range from the continuing promulgation of relatively simple messages to the more complex and demanding task of understanding, enabling and encouraging negotiation. The growing sophistication of many men's strategies needs to be encouraged, while remembering the needs of those who are new to sex.

Such initiatives need to be informed by and to work within a theory of sex and sexuality. The single focus of HIV prevention runs the risk of elevating the need for safer sex to a level which negates the real process of sexual pleasure. Some HIV professionals run the risk of being blinded by their own evangelism and condemning where encouragement is more appropriate. In this book we have sought to do just this: to try to isolate within the practice of sex those elements which are central to an understanding of risk behaviour.

The agenda of HIV prevention for gay and bisexual men in the coming years is intricate and complex. There is a need not only to develop and sustain programs which address these disparate needs, itself a challenge in a health care system which has, as we have noted, sought to distance itself from the needs of gay men. Also there is a need to coordinate these programs, recognising that some agencies will have strengths where others are weak. Thus, for example, the Health Education Authority (HEA) with its expertise and background in this area, appears well able to mount large-scale national campaigns, which could be used to put over messages of relatively simple content. The HEA is rather less suited, both because it is based in London and because of its problematic relationship with the government, to establishing local programs of group work or peer education (though we recognise their funding of the MESMAC projects which provide pilot projects of this sort). These are, presumably, best managed by local groups specialised in low level, small-scale focused interventions which take account of the specific needs of the local community.

It would be a mistake, however, to assume that every local District HIV Prevention Coordinator (DHPC) is as willing or capable of initiating such programs. In the traditional British fashion AIDS organisations in this country have grown up in a haphazard and uncoordinated manner. In this diversity is the source of great strength and innovation. As HIV becomes increasingly normalised within the health care system, and the contract culture of the new National Health Service is weighted against prophylactic medicine of all kinds, there may be a case for an authoritative coordinating body which would act as a means of disseminating good practice and as a lobbying organisation near the heart of government.

There are those who have seen in the Australian National Council on AIDS a model of this sort of organisation. Whether such an organisation would work in the more conservative British context must remain unclear, though previous attempts have, as we have noted in Chapter 3, not been successful. It is also most probable that any such organisation would downplay the needs of gay men, along with drug users and other marginal groups, since it would, almost by definition, be composed of figures acceptable to the establishment. Rather, it seems more likely that an organisation from within the gay communities themselves would be more valuable. It remains to be seen whether the recently founded Gay Men Fighting AIDS (GMFA) will come to assume such a role. It seems to us, however, that to do so, it needs to encourage a diversity of response and opinion rather than to impose a strictly separatist criterion of political correctness on individuals, initiatives and organisations.

The future remains uncertain as we continue to wait for the medical scientists to live up to their own propaganda and achieve the breakthrough they have promised for the last eight years or so. Into that uncertainty we must project our best efforts to understand the processes of safer sex. To that end we have produced this volume.

References

ADAM, B. (1987) *The Rise of a Gay and Lesbian Movement*, Twayne, Boston.

ADIB, S.M., JOSEPH, J.G., OSTROW, D.G., TAL, M. and SCHWARTZ, S.A. (1991) *Relapse in Sexual Behaviour among Homosexual Men: a 2-year Follow-up from the Chicago MACS/CCS*, AIDS, 5, pp. 757–60.

AGGLETON, P. (1989) Evaluating Health Education about AIDS, in AGGLETON, P., DAVIES, P. and HART, G. (Eds) *AIDS: Social Representations, Social Practices*, Falmer Press, London, pp. 220–36.

AGGLETON, P., COXON, A.P.M. and WEATHERBURN, P. (1990) *AIDS Health Promotion Activities Directed Towards Gay and Bisexual Men in London (UK)*, A briefing document prepared for the World Health Organization Global Programme on AIDS.

AJZEN, I. and MADDEN, T.J. (1986) Prediction of Goal-Directed Behavior: Attitudes, Intentions and Perceived Behavioral Control, *Journal of Experimental Social Psychology*, 22, pp. 453–474.

ALCORN, K. (1988) Illness, Metaphor and AIDS, in AGGLETON, P. and HOMANS, H. (Ed.) *Social Aspects of AIDS*, Falmer Press, Lewes, pp. 83–105.

ALTMAN, D. (1971) *Homosexual Oppression and Liberation*, Outerbridge & Dienstfry, New York.

ALTMAN, D. (1986) *AIDS and the New Puritanism*, Pluto, London.

BANDURA, A. (1977) Self-Efficacy: Toward a Unifying Theory of Behavioural Change, *Psychological Review*, 84, pp. 191–215.

BARBADETTE, G. (1982) *The Social Triumph of the Sexual Will: A Conversation with Michel Foucault*, (tr. Lemon B) Christopher Street, 6, 4, pp. 36–41.

BARRINGTON, J.S. (1981) *Sexual Alternatives for Men: Facts and Fantasies* (Vol. 1), The Alternative Publishing Co., London.

BARTHOLOMEW, D.J. (1982) *Stochastic Processes for Social Processes*, Wiley, London.

BARTLETT, N. (1988) *Who Was That Man*, Serpents Tail, London.

BAXTER, D. (1990) *Maintenance of Safe Sex Norms in the Gay Community*, Paper presented at the IVth Australian National AIDS Conference, Canberra.

BECKER, M.H. (Ed.) (1974) Health Education Monograph, 2, 4, special edition on the HBM, reprinted as *The Health Belief Model and Personal Health Behaviour*, Charles Black, New Jersey.

BELL, A.P. and WEINBERG, M.S. (1978) *Homosexualities: A Study of Diversity Among Men and Women*, Simon and Schuster, New York.

BENNETT, G., CHAPMAN, S., and BRAY, F. (1989) A Potential Source for the Transmission of the Human Immunodeficiency Virus into the Heterosexual Population: Bisexual Men Who Frequent 'Beats', *Medical Journal of Australia*, 151, pp. 314–18.

BERGLER, E. (1956) *Homosexuality: Disease or Way of Life?*, Collier-MacMillan, New York.

BERKOWITZ, S.D. (1982) *An Introduction to Structural Analysis*, London, Butterworth.

BERLIN, I. Two Concepts of Liberty, reprinted in QUINTON, A. (Ed.), *Political Philosophy*, pp. 141–52, OUP, Oxford.

BERRIDGE, V. (1992) AIDS, the Media and Health Policy, in AGGLETON, P., DAVIES, P.M. and HART, G. (Eds) *AIDS: Rights, Risk and Reason*, Falmer Press, London, pp. 13–27.

BÉRUBÉ, A. (1983) Marching to a Different Drummer, reprinted in DUBERMAN, M.B., VICINIUS, M. and CHAUNCEY, G. (Eds) (1991) *Hidden from History*, Penguin, London.

BIEBER, I., DAIN, H.J., DINCE, P.R. *et al.* (1962) *Homosexuality: A Psychoanalytic Study of Male Homosexuals*, Basic Books, Random House, New York.

BIRCH, K. (1980) The Politics of Autonomy in Gay Left Collective (Eds) *Homosexuality: Power and Politics*, Alison and Busby, London, pp. 85–92.

BLASBAND, D. and PEPLAU, L.A. (1985) Sexual Exclusivity Versus Openness in Gay Male Couples, *Archives of Sexual Behaviour*, 145, pp. 395–412.

BLUMSTEIN, P. and SCHWARTZ, P. (1983) *American Couples*, William Morrow, New York.

BLUMSTEIN, P. and SCHWARTZ, P. (1976) *Bisexuality in Men*, Urban Life, 5, pp. 339–58.

BOCHOW, M. (1991) Le Safer Sex, 'Une Discussion Sans Fin': Quelques Remarques au Sujet de la Discussion Actuelle, to appear in M. POLLAK (Ed.).

BOCHOW, M. (1990) *AIDS and Gay Men: Individual Strategies and Collective Coping*, European Sociological Review, 6, 2, pp. 181–188.

BOLTON, R., VINCKE, J. and MAK, R. (1992) *Gay Saunas: Venues of HIV Transmission or AIDS Prevention?*, poster presented at VIII International Conference on AIDS, Amsterdam, PoD 5172.

BOULTON, M. and WEATHERBURN, P. (1990) *Literature Review on Bisexuality and HIV Transmission*, Report commissioned by the Social and Behavioural Research Unit, Global Programme on AIDS, World Health Organisation.

BOULTON, M., SCHRAMM EVANS, Z., FITZPATRICK, R. and HART, G. (1990) Bisexual Men: Women, Safer Sex and HIV Infection, in AGGLETON, P., DAVIES, P.M., and HART, G. *AIDS: Responses, Interventions and Care*, Falmer Press, London, pp. 65–78.

BRAY, A. (1982) *Homosexuality in Renaissance England*, Gay Men's Press, London.

BROWN, P. (1988) *The Body and Society: Men, Women and Sexual Renunciation in Early Christianity*, Faber, London.

BUBER, M. (1970) *I and Thou*, T. & T. Clark, Edinburgh.

BULLOUGH, V.L. (1974) Homosexuality and the Medical Model, *Journal of Homosexuality*, 1, 1, pp. 99–110.

CAHILL, K.M. (Ed.) (1983) *The AIDS Epidemic*, London, Hutchinson.

CANAVAN, P. (1984) The Gay Community at Jacob Riis Park, in BOGGS, V. (Ed.). *The Apple Sliced*, Berger & Garvey, South Hadley, MA.

CARNE, C., WELLER, I. and JOHNSON, A. *et al.* (1987) *Prevalence of Antibodies to Human Immunodeficiency Virus, Gonorrhoea Rates and Changed Sexual Behaviour in Homosexual Men in London*, Lancet, i, pp. 656–8.

CARRIER, J.M. (1976) *Cultural Factors Affecting Urban Mexican Male Homosexual Behaviour*, Archives of Sexual Behaviour, 5, 2, pp. 103–124.

CARRIER, J.M. (1977) *Sex-Role Preference as an Explanatory Variable in Homosexual Behaviour*, Archives of Sexual Behaviour, 6, 1, pp. 53–65.

CARRIER, J.M. (1971) *Sex-role Preference as an Explanatory Variable in Homosexual Behaviour*, Archives of Sexual Behaviour, 6, 1, pp. 53–65.

CARRIER, J.M. (1971) *Participants in Urban Mexican Male Homosexual Encounters*, Archives of Sexual Behaviour, 1, 4, pp. 279–291.

CASS, V.C. (1984) Homosexual Identity Formation: Testing a Theoretical Model, *Journal of Sex Research*, 20, pp. 143–67.

CATANIA, J.A., KEGELES, S.M. and COATES, T.J. (1990) Towards an Understanding of Risk Behaviour: The CAPS AIDS Risk Reduction Model (ARRM), *Health Education Quarterly*, 17, 1, pp. 53–72.

CDC (Centers for Disease Control), (1986) Additional Recommendations to Reduce Sexual and Drug Abuse Related Transmission of HTLVIII/LAV, *Mortality and Morbidity Weekly Report*, 35, pp. 152–155.

CHESSER, E. (1959) *Odd Man Out*, Gollancz, London.

CHMIEL, J.S., DETELS, R., KASLOW, R.A. *et al.* (1987) Factors Associated with Prevalent Human Immunodeficiency Virus (HIV) Infection in the Multicenter AIDS Cohort Study, *American Journal of Epidemiology*, 126, pp. 568–577.

COATES, R., CALZAVARA, L., SOSKOLNE, C. *et al.* (1988) Validity of Sexual Histories in a Prospective Study of Male Sexual Contacts of Men with AIDS or an AIDS Related Condition, *American Journal of Epidemiology*, 78, pp. 1535–8.

COCHRAN, W.G., MOSTELLER, F. and TUKEY, J.W. (1954) Statistical Problems of the Kinsey Report, *Journal of the American Statistical Association*, 48, pp. 673–716.

COHEN, S. (1980) *Folk Devils and Moral Panics: The Creation of the Mods and Rockers*, (2nd ed.), Martin Robertson, Oxford.

CONANT, M., HARDY, D., SERNATINGER, J., SPICER, D., and LEVY, J.A. (1986) Condoms Prevent Transmission of AIDS-Associated Retrovirus, *Journal of the American Medical Association*, 255, p. 1706.

CONNELL, R.W., CRAWFORD, J., KIPPAX, S., DOWSETT, G.W., BAXTER, D., WATSON, L. and BERG, R. (1989) Facing the Epidemic: Changes in the Sexual Lives of Gay and Bisexual Men in Australia and Their Implications for AIDS Prevention Strategies, *Social Problems*, 36, 4, pp. 384–402.

CONNELL, R.W. and KIPPAX, S. (1990) Sexuality in the AIDS Crisis: Patterns of Sexual Practice and Pleasure in a Sample of Australian Gay and Bisexual Men, *Journal of Sex Research*, 27, 2, pp. 167–196.

CONNELL, R.W., CRAWFORD, J., KIPPAX, S., DOWSETT, G.W., BOND, G., BAXTER, D., BERG, R. and WATSON, L. (1988) *Social Aspects of the Prevention of AIDS: Study A, Report No.1 Method and Sample*, Macquarie University, Sydney.

CONNOR, S. and S. KINGMAN (1988) *The search for the Virus: The Scientific Discovery of AIDS and the Quest for a Cure*, Harmondsworth, Penguin.

COOMBS, C.H. (1964) *A Theory of Data*, New York, Wiley.

CORY, D.W. and LEROY, J.P. (1963) *The Homosexual and His Society: A View From Within*, Citadel, London.

CORY, D.W. (1953) *The Homosexual Outlook: A Subjective Approach*, Peter Nevill, London.

CORZINE, J. and KIRBY, R. (1977) Cruising The Truckers: Sexual Encounters in a Highway Rest Area, *Urban Life*, 6, pp. 171–92.

COTTON, T. and KUMARI, V. (1990) Local Authorities and HIV-Related Illness, in AGGLETON, P., DAVIES, P.M. and HART, G. (Eds) *AIDS: Individual, Cultural and Policy Dimensions*, Falmer Press, London, pp. 213–19.

COXON, A.P.M., DAVIES, P.M., HUNT, A., MCMANUS, T.J., REES, C., WEATHERBURN, P. and HICKSON, F.C.I. (1993) Strategies in Eliciting Sensitive, Sexual Information: The Case of Gay Men, *Sociological Review*, [in press].

COXON, A.P.M., DAVIES, P.M., HUNT, A.J., WEATHERBURN, P., MCMANUS, T.J. and REES, C. (1992) The Structure of Sexual Behaviour, *Journal of Sex Research*, 29, 1, pp. 61–83.

COXON, A.P.M. (1988) 'Something Sensational ...'. The Sexual Diary as a Tool for Mapping Detailed Sexual Behaviour, *Sociological Review*, 36, 2, pp. 353–367.

COXON, A.P.M. (1986) *Report of Pilot Study: Project on Sexual Lifestyles of Non-Heterosexual Males*, Project SIGMA Working Paper no. 1, SRU, University College, Cardiff.

CRANE, P. (1981) *Gays and the Law*, Pluto, London.

CRIMP, D. (1989) *AIDS: Cultural Analysis, Cultural Activism*, MIT Press, Cambridge, MA.

D'EMILIO, J.D. (1983) *Sexual Politics, Sexual Communities: The Making of a Homosexual Minority in the United States 1940–1970*, University of Chicago Press, Chicago.

DARROW, W.W., ECHENBERG, D.F., JAFFE, H.W., O'MALLEY, P.M., BYERS, R.H., GETCHELL, J.P. and CURRAN, J.W. (1987) Risk Factors for Human Immunodeficiency Virus (HIV) Infections in Homosexual Men, *American Journal of Public Health*, 77, 4, pp. 479–483

DAVIES, P.M. and COXON, A.P.M. (1990) Patterns in Homosexual Behaviour: Use of the Diary Method, in HUBERT, M. (Ed.), *Sexual Behaviour and Risks of HIV Infection*, Facultés Universitaires Saint-Louis, Brussels.

DAVIES, P.M. and WEATHERBURN, P. (1991) Towards a General Model of Sexual Negotiation, in AGGLETON, P., DAVIES, P. and HART, G. (Eds) *AIDS: Responses, Interventions and Care*, Falmer Press, Lewes, pp. 111–25.

DAVIES, P.M., WEATHERBURN, P., HUNT, A.J., HICKSON, F.C.I., MCMANUS, T.J. and COXON, A.P.M. (1992) The Sexual Behaviour of Young, Gay Men in England and Wales, *AIDS Care*, 4, 3, pp. 259–272.

DAVIES, P. (1992) On Relapse: Recidivism or Rational Response?, in AGGLETON, P., DAVIES, P. and HART, G., *AIDS: Rights, Risk and Reason*, Falmer, London, pp. 133–41.

DAVIES, P.M. and SIMPSON, P. (1990) On Male Homosexual Prostitution and HIV, in AGGLETON, P., DAVIES, P.M. and HART, G. (Eds) *AIDS: Individual, Cultural and Social Perspectives*, Falmer Press, London, pp. 103–19.

DAVIES, P.M. (1986) *Some Problems in Defining and Sampling Non-Heterosexual Males*, Project SIGMA Working Paper 3, London.

Davies, P.M. (1989) Some Notes on the Structure of Sexual Acts, in Aggleton, P., Davies, P. and Hart, G. (Eds) *AIDS: Social Representations, Social Practices*, Falmer Press, London, pp. 147–59.

Davies, P.M., Hunt, A.J., Macourt, M.P.A. and Weatherburn, P. (1990) *Longitudinal Study of the Sexual Behaviour of Homosexual Males under the Impact of AIDS: A Final Report to the Department of Health*, Project SIGMA, London.

Davies, P.M. (1990) *Patterns in Homosexual Relations: the Use of the Diary Method*, Project SIGMA Working Paper no. 17, London.

Delph, E.W. (1978) *The Silent Community: Public Homosexual Encounters*, Sage, Beverley Hills CA.

Department of Health/Welsh Office (1988) *Short-term Prediction of HIV Infection and AIDS in England and Wales: Report of a Working Group*, HMSO, London.

Detels, R., Fahey, J.F., Schwartz, K., Greene, R.S., Visscher, B.R. and Gottlieb, M.S. (1983) *Relations Between Sexual Practices and T-cell Subsets in Homosexually Active Men*, Lancet, 1, pp. 1034–9.

Douglas, M. (1966) *Purity and Danger: An Analysis of the Concepts of Pollution and Taboo*, Routledge and Kegan Paul, London.

Dover, K.J. (1978) *Greek Homosexuality*, Harvard University Press, Cambridge, MA.

Dowsett, G., Davis, M. and Connell, B. (1992) Gay Men, HIV/AIDS and Social Research: An Antipodean Perspective, in Aggleton, P., Davies, P.M. and Hart, G. (Eds) *AIDS: Rights, Risk and Reason*, Falmer, London, pp. 1–12.

Dworkin, A. (1987) *Intercourse*, Martin Secker & Warburg Ltd., London.

Ekstrand, M., Stall, R., Marlett, A., Pollack, L., McKusick, L. and Coates, T. (1992) *Frequent and Infrequent Relapsers Need Different AIDS Prevention Programs*, poster Presented at VIIIth International Conference on AIDS, Amsterdam, PoD 5129.

Ekstrand, M.L., Stall, R.D., Coates, T.J. and McKusick, L. (1989) *Risky Sex Relapse, the Next Challenge for AIDS Prevention Programs*, the AIDS Behavioural Research Project Paper presented at Vth International Conference on AIDS, Montreal, T.D.O.8.

Ekstrand, M.L., Coates, T.J., Guydish, J.R., Hauck, W.W., Collete, M.S., Hulley, S.B. (1992) *Bisexual Men in San Francisco Are Not a Common Vector for Spreading HIV Infection to Women; The San Francisco Men's Health Study*, Unpublished Manuscript.

Ellis, H.H. with Symonds, J.A. (1897) *Sexual Inversion*, Wilson Macmillan, London.

Ellman, R. (1987) *Oscar Wilde*, Penguin, Harmondsworth.

Emmons, C.A., Joseph, J.G., Kessler, R.C., Wortman, C.B., Montgomery, S.B. and Ostrow, D.G. (1986) Psycholosocial Predictors of Reported Behaviour Change in Homosexual Men at Risk from AIDS, *Health Education Quarterly*, 13, 4, pp. 331–345.

European Study Group (1989) Risk Factors for Male to Female Transmission of HIV, *British Medical Journal*, 298, pp. 411–414.

Evans, B.A., McLean, K.A., Dawson, S.G. *et al.* (1989) Trends in Sexual Behaviour and Risk Factors for HIV Infection among Homosexual Men 1984–7, *British Medical Journal*, 298, pp. 215–8.

Evans, B.A., McCormack, S.M., Bond, R.A. *et al.* (1988) Human Immunodeficiency Virus Infection, Hepatitis B Infection and Sexual Behaviour of Women Attending a Genito-urinary Medicine Clinic, *British Medical Journal*, 296, pp. 473–75.

Farquhar, C. (1991) Answering Children's Questions about HIV/AIDS in the Primary School: Are Teachers Prepared?, in Aggleton, P., Davies, P.M. and Hart, G. *AIDS: Responses, Interventions and Care*, Falmer Press, London, pp. 191–211.

Fitzpatrick, R., Boulton, M. and Hart, G. (1989) Gay Men's Sexual Behaviour in Response to AIDS, in Aggleton, P., Davies, P. and Hart, G. (Eds) (1989) *AIDS: Social Representations, Social Practices*, Falmer Press, London, pp. 127–46.

Fitzpatrick, R., Boulton, M. and Hart, G. (1990) Variation in Sexual Behaviour in Gay Men, in Aggleton, P., Davies, P. and Hart, G. (Eds) (1990) *AIDS: Individual, Cultural and Policy Dimensions*, Falmer, London, pp. 121–32.

Fitzpatrick, R., Boulton, M., Hart, G., Dawson, J. and McLean, J. (1989) High Risk Sexual Behaviour and Condom Use in a Sample of Homosexual and Bisexual Men, *Health Trends*, 21, pp. 76–79.

Fitzpatrick, R., Hart, G., Boulton, M., McLean, J. and Dawson, J. (1989) Heterosexual Sexual Behaviour in a Sample of Homosexually Active Males, *Genito-Urinary Medicine, 1989*; 65, pp. 259–62.

Fitzpatrick, M. and Milligan, D. (1987) *The Truth about the AIDS Panic*, Junius Press, London.

Foege, W. (1983) The National Pattern of AIDS, in Cahill, K.M. (Ed.), *The AIDS Epidemic*, Hutchinson, London, pp. 7–17.

Foucault, M. (1985) *The Use of Pleasure: History of Sexuality Volume Two*, Random House, New York.

Foucault, M. (1982/3) *Sexual Act, Sexual Choice*, an interview with Michel Foucault by James O'Higgins, Salmagundi, 58/9, pp. 10–24.

Foucault, M. (1976) *La Volonté de Savoir*, Éditions Gallimar, Paris. (tr. Hurley R, 1979: *The History of Sexuality: An Introduction*; Allen Lane, London.

Fox, R., Ostrow, D.G. and Valdiserri, R.O. *et al.* (1987) *Changes in Sexual Activities Among Participants in Multicenter AIDS Cohort Study*, III International Conference on AIDS, Washington, DC.

Frankenberg, R. (1989) One Epidemic or Three? Cultural, Social and Historical Aspects of the AIDS Pandemic, in Aggleton, P., Davies, P. and Hart, G. (Eds) (1989) *AIDS: Social Representations, Social Practices*; Falmer, London, pp. 21–38.

Freeman, R. (1992) The Politics of AIDS in Britain and Germany, in Aggleton, P., Davies, P. and Hart, G. (Eds) (1992) *AIDS: Rights, Risk and Reason*, Falmer Press, London, pp. 53–67.

Frutchey, C. and Williams, A.M. (1992) *Cultural Factors in Gay Male Group Sexual Interactions: Findings and Implications for Planning HIV Prevention Strategies*, poster presented at VIII International Conference on AIDS, Amsterdam, PoD 5181.

Fulford, K.W., Catterall, R.D., Hoinville, E., Lim, K.S. and Wilson, G.D. (1983) Social and Psychological Characteristics in the Distribution of Male Clinic Attenders, *British Journal of Venereal Diseases*, 596, pp. 386–93.

Galtung, J. (1967) *Theory and Methods of Social Research*, Allen and Unwin, London.

Gilbert, A.N. (1981) Conceptions of Homosexuality and Sodomy in Western History, *Journal of Homosexuality*, 6, 1/2, pp. 57–68.

GILBERT, N. (1982) *Modelling Society*, Allen and Unwin, London.

GILMAN, S. (1988) *Disease and Representation*, Cornell University Press, London.

GOEDERT, J.J., SARNGADHARAN, M.G., BIGGAR, R.J., WEISS, S.H., WINN, D.M., GROSSMAN, R.J., GREENE, M.H., BODNER, A.J., MANN, D.L., STRONG, D.M., GALLO, R.C. and BLATTNER, W.A. (1984) *Determinants of Retrovirus (HTLV-III) Antibody and Immunodeficiency Conditions in Homosexual Men*, The Lancet, 2, pp. 711–716.

GOEDERT, J.J., BIGGAR, R.J., WINN, D.M., MANN, D.L., BYAR, D.P., STRONG, D.M. *et al.* (1985) Decreased Helper T Lymphocytes in Homosexual Men. II Sexual Practices, *American Journal of Epidemiology*, 121, pp. 637–344.

GOFFMAN, E. (1968) *The Presentation of Self in Everyday Life*, Pelican, London.

GOLD, R., SKINNER, M., GRANT, P. and PLUMMER, D. (1989) *Situational Factors Associated with and Rationalisations Employed to Justify Unprotected Intercourse in Gay Men*, paper presented at the Vth International Conference on AIDS, Montreal, T.D.O.7.

GOLDSTEIN, R. (1989) AIDS and the Social Contract, in CARTER, E. and WATNEY, S. (Eds) *Taking Liberties: AIDS and Cultural Politics*, Serpent's Tail, London.

GOLOMBOK, S., SKETCHLEY, J. and RUST, J. (1989) Condom Use Among Homosexual Men, *AIDS Care*, 1, 1, pp. 27–33.

GOTTLIEB, M.S., SCHROFF, R., SCHANKER, H.M. and WEISMAN, D.O. *et al.* (1981) Pneumocystis Carinii Pneumonia and Mucosal Candiasis in Previously Health Homosexual Men: Evidence of a New Acquired Cellular Immunodeficiency, *New England Journal of Medicine*, 305, 24, pp. 1425–31.

GROOPMAN, J., MAYER, K., SARNGADHARAN, M., AYOTTE, D., DEVICO, A., FINSBERG, R., SLISKI, A. and ALLAN, J.D. (1985) Seroepidemiology of Human T-Lymphotropic Virus Type III Among Homosexual Men with Acquired Immuno-deficiency Syndrome or Generalized Lymphadenopathy and among Asymptomatic Controls in Boston, *Annals of Internal Medicine*, 102, pp. 334–337.

GROSSKURTH, P. (1980) *Havelock Ellis*, AA Knopf, New York.

GROVER, J.Z. (1989) AIDS: Keywords, in CRIMP, D. (Ed.), *AIDS: Cultural Analysis, Cultural Activism*, MIT Press, Cambridge, MA

HAEBERLE, E.J. (1981) Swastika, Pink Triangle and Yellow Star — the Destruction of Sexology and the Persecution of Homosexuals in Nazi Germany, *The Journal of Sex Research*, 17, 3, pp. 270–287.

HALL-CARPENTER ARCHIVES (1989) *Walking After Midnight; Gay Men's Life Stories*, Routledge, London.

HALL-CARPENTER ARCHIVES (1989) *Inventing Ourselves; Lesbian Life Stories*, Routledge, London.

HALPERIN, D.M. (1989) Sex before Sexuality: Pederasty, Politics and Power in Classical Athens, in DUBERMAN, M.B., VICINIUS, M. and CHAUNCEY, G. (Eds), *Hidden from History: Reclaiming the Gay and Lesbian Past*, New American Library, New York, pp. 37–53.

HAMMERSMITH, S.K. and WEINBERG, M.S. (1973) *Homosexual Identity: Commitment, Adjustment and Significant Others*, Sociometry, 36, pp. 56–79.

HANSARD, 124(65), Col.1001. 15 December 1987.

HARRIS, M. (1973) *The Dilly Boys: Male Prostitutes in Picadilly*, Croom Helm, London.

HARRY, J. and DE VALL, W.B. (1978) *The Social Organisation of Gay Males*, Praeger, New York.

HARRY, J. (1976) On the Validity of Typologies of Gay Males, *Journal of Homosexuality*, 2, pp. 143–52.

HART, G., MCCLEAN, J., BOULTON, M., DAWSON, J. and FITZPATRICK, R. (1991) *Maintenance and Change in Safer Sex Behaviours in a Cohort of Gay Men in England*, paper presented to the VIIth International Conference on AIDS, Florence; W.D.4139.

HAUSER, R. (1962) *The Homosexual Society*, Bodley Head, London.

HERDT, G., LEAP, W. and SOVINE, M. (1991) Anthropology, Sex and AIDS, *Journal of Sex Research*, 28, 2, (special issue).

HICKSON, F.C.I, DAVIES, P.M., HUNT, A.J., WEATHERBURN, P., MCMANUS, T.J. and COXON, A.P.M. (1992) *Maintenance of Open, Gay Relationships, Strategies Against For Protection HIV Infection*, AIDS Care, 4, 4, [in press].

HICKSON, F. (1991) *Sexual Exclusivity, Non-Exclusivity and HIV*, Project SIGMA Working No. Paper 31, London.

HILLIER, H.C. (1988) Estimation of HIV Prevalence in England and Wales — the Direct Approach, in Department of Health/Welsh Office, *Short Term Prediction of HIV Infection and AIDS in England and Wales*, HMSO, London, pp. 48–52.

HIRSCHFELD, M. (1920) *Die Homosexualität des Mannes und des Weibes*, L. Marcus Verlagbuchhandlung, Berlin.

HOFF, C.C., MCKUSICK, L., HILLIARD, B., EKSTRAND, M. and COATES, T.J. (1992) *Changes in Gay Relationships Before the AIDS Epidemic and Now*, poster presented at the VIIIth International Conference on AIDS, Amsterdam, PoD 5186.

HOMANS, H. and AGGLETON, P. (1988) Health Education, HIV Infection and AIDS, in HOMANS, H. and AGGLETON, P. (Eds), *Social Aspects of AIDS*, Falmer Press, London, pp. 154–76.

HOME OFFICE/SCOTTISH HOME DEPARTMENT (1957) *Report of the Committee on Homosexual Offenses and Prostitution*, Cmnd 247, HMSO, London.

HOOKER, E. (1965) *An Empirical Study of Some Relations Between Sexual Patterns and Gender Identity in Male Homosexuals*, in *Sex Research: New Developments*, Holt, New York, 1965, pp. 24–25.

HORTON, M. (1989) Bugs, Drugs and Placebos: The Opulence of Truth, or How to Make a Treatment Decision in an Epidemic, in CARTER, E. and WATNEY, S. (Eds), *Taking Liberties: AIDS and Cultural Politics*, Serpent's Tail, London.

HUME, D. (1974) *A Treatise on Human Nature*, (2 vols) Everyman, London.

HUMPHREYS, L. (1972) *Out of the Closets*, Prentice-Hall, Englewood Cliffs, NJ.

HUMPHREYS, L. (1970) *Tearoom Trade: Impersonal Sex in Public Places*, Aldine, Chicago.

HUNT, A.J., DAVIES, P.M., MCMANUS, T.J., WEATHERBURN, P., HICKSON, F.C.I., CHRISTOFINIS, G., COXON, A.P.M. and SUTHERLAND, S. (1992) *HIV-1 Infection In A Cohort of Gay and Bisexual Men*, BMJ, 305, pp. 561–2.

HUNT, A.J., WEATHERBURN, P., HICKSON, F.C.I., DAVIES, P.M., MCMANUS, T.J. and COXON, A.P.M. (1993) *Changes in Condom Use by Gay Men*, AIDS Care [in press].

HUNT, A.J., CONNELL, J., CHRISTOFINIS, G., PARRY, J.V., WEATHERBURN, P., HICKSON, F.C.I., COXON, A.P.M., DAVIES, P.M., MCMANUS, T.J. and SUTHERLAND, S. (1993) *The Testing of Saliva Samples For HIV-1 Antibodies: Reliability in a Non-Clinic Setting*, Genitourinary Medicine, [in press].

Hunt, A.J., Coxon, A.P.M., Davies, P.M., Weatherburn, P. and McManus, T.J. (1991b) *Changes in Sexual Behaviour in a Large Cohort of Homosexually Active Men in England and Wales 1988–1989*, BMJ, 302, pp. 505–6.

Hunt, A.J., Davies, P.M., Weatherburn, P., Coxon, A.P.M. and McManus, T.J. (1991a) *Sexual Partners, Penetrative Sexual Partners and HIV Risk*, AIDS 5, pp. 723–28.

Hunt, A.J., Christofinis, G., Coxon, A.P.M., Davies, P.M., McManus, T.J., Sutherland, S. and Weatherburn, P. (1990) *Seroprevalence of HIV-1 Infection in a Cohort of Homosexually Active Men*, Genitourinary Medicine 66, pp. 423–27.

Hunt, A.J. and Davies, P.M. (1990) What is a Sexual Encounter?, in Aggleton, P., Davies, P.M. and Hart, G. (Eds), *AIDS: Responses, Interventions and Care*, Falmer Press, London.

Huusen, A.H. (1989) Sodomy in the Dutch Republic During the Eighteenth Century, in Duberman, M.B., Vicinius, M. and Chauncey, G. (Eds), *Hidden from History: Reclaiming the Gay and Lesbian Past*, New American Library, New York, pp. 141–152.

Jay, K. and Young, A. (1979) *The Gay Report: Lesbians and Gay Men Speak Out About Their Sexual Experiences and Lifestyles*, Summit Books, New York.

Jeffery-Poulter, S. (1991) *Peers, Queers and Commons: The Struggle for Gay Law Reform from 1950 to the Present*, Routledge, London.

Jeffries, E., Willoughby, K.B. and Boyko, W. *et al.* (1985) The Vancouver Lymphadenopathy-AIDS Study 2: Seroepidemiology of HTLV-III Antibody, *Canadian Medical Association Journal*, 132, pp. 1373–1377.

Jellinek, E.M. (1960) *The Disease Concept of Alcoholism*, Hillhouse, New Haven, Conn.

Johnson, A.M. and Laga, M. (1988) *Heterosexual Transmission of HIV*, AIDS, 2 (suppl. 1) S49–S56.

Johnson, A.M., Parry, J.V., Best, S.J., Smith, A.M., De Silva, M. and Mortimer, P.P. (1988) *HIV Surveillance by Testing Saliva*, AIDS 2, pp. 369–371.

Joseph, *et al.* (1987) *Magnitude and Determinants of Behavioural Risk Reduction: Longitudinal Analysis of a Cohort at Risk from AIDS*, Psychology and Health 1, pp. 73–96.

Kahneman, D. and Tversky, A. (1972) Subjective Probability: A judgement of Representatives, *Cognitive Psychology*, 3, pp. 430–454.

Kameny, F. (1969) Gay is Good, in Weltge, R. (Ed.), *The Same Sex*, Pilgrim, Philadelphia.

Katz, J. (1976) *Gay American History; Lesbians and Gay Men in the USA*, Crowell, New York.

Kegebein, V., Bense, B. and Wohlfeiler, D. (1992) *Keeping San Francisco Sex Clubs Open and Safe: Community/Public Health Partnerships*, poster presented at VIII International Conference on AIDS, Amsterdam, PoD 5128.

Kennedy, H. (1988) *Ulrichs: The Life and Works of Karl Heinrich Ulrichs, Pioneer of the Modern Gay Movement*, Alyson, Boston.

Kennedy, H. (1981) The 'Third Sex' Theory of Karl Heinrich Ulrichs, *Journal of Homosexuality*, 6, pp. 130–11.

KEOGH, P., CHURCH, J., VEARNALS, S. and GREEN, J. (1992) *Investigation of Motivational and Behavioural Factors Influencing Men Who Have Sex With Men in Public Toilets Cottaging*, poster presented at VIIIth International Conference on AIDS, Amsterdam, PoD 5187.

KING, E., ROONEY, M. and SCOTT, P. (1992) 'HIV Prevention for Gay Men: A Survey of Initiatives in the UK', North West Thames Regional Health Authority HIV Project.

KINGSLEY, L.A., DETELS, R., KASLOW, R., POLK, B.F., RINALDO, C.R., CHMIEL, J., DETRE, K., KESLEY, S.F., ODAKA, N., OSTROW, D., VAN RADEN, M. and VISSCHER, B. (1987) 'Risk Factors for Seroconversion to Human Immunodeficiency Virus among Male Homosexuals', *The Lancet*, 14 February, pp. 345–348.

KINSEY, A.C., POMEROY, W.B., MARTIN, C.E. and GEBHARD, P.H. (1953) *Sexual Behaviour in the Human Female*, Saunders, Philadelphia.

KINSEY, A.C. (1942) *Isolating Mechanisms in the Gall Wasp*, Biol. Symposia, 6.

KINSEY, A.C., POMEROY, W.B. and MARTIN, C.E. (1948) *Sexual Behaviour in the Human Male*, WB Saunders, Philadelphia.

KIPPAX, S., DOWSETT, G.W., DAVIS, M., RODDEN, P. and CRAWFORD, J. (1992) *Sustaining safe Sex or Relapse: Gay Men's Response to HIV*, paper presented at the VIIIth International Conference on AIDS, Amsterdam, TuD 0545.

KIPPAX, S. *et al.* (1990) *The Importance of Gay Community in the Prevention of HIV Transmission: A Case Study of Australian Men Who Have Sex With Men*, Social Aspects of the Prevention of AIDS Project, Report no. 7, Macquarrie University, Sydney.

KOCHEMS, L.M. (1987) *Meanings and Health Implications: Gay Men's Sexuality*, Paper presented at the American Anthropological Association.

KOSOFSKY-SEDGWICK, E. (1991) *Epistemology of the Closet*, Harvester Wheatsheaf, New York.

KRAFFT-EBING, R. VON (1925) *Psychopathia Sexualis with special reference to the Antipathic Sexual Instinct: A Medico-Forensic Study*, (tr. REBMAN, F.J.), Physicians and Surgeons Book Co., New York.

KRAMER, L. (1978) *Faggots*, Random House, New York.

LAHR, J. (Ed.) (1986) *The Orton Diaries*, Methuen, London.

LANCASTER, R.N. (1988) 'Subject Honour and Object Shame: The Construction of Male Homosexuality and Stigma in Nicaragua', *Ethnology*, 27, 2, pp. 111–125.

LEE, J.A. (1988) 'Forbidden Colours of Love: Patterns of Gay Love and Gay Liberation', in DECECCO, J.P. (Ed.), *Gay Relationships*, Harrington Park Press, London.

MACINTYRE, A. (1973) 'The Idea of a Social Science', in RYAN, A. (Ed.) *The Philosophy of Social Explanation*, 15–32; OUP, London.

MAGEE, B. (1966) *One in Twenty*, Secker and Warburg, London.

MARMOR, M., FRIEDMAN-KEIN, A., ZOLLER-PAZNER, S., STAHL, R.E., RUBINSTEIN, P., LAUBENSTEIN, L., WILLIAMS, D.C., KLEIN, R.J. and SPIGLAND, I. (1984) 'Kaposi's Sarcoma in Homosexual Men', *Annals of Internal Medicine*, 100, pp. 809–815.

MAROTTA, T. (1981) *The Politics of Homosexuality*, Houghton Mifflin, Boston.

MARTIN, J.L. (1987) *The Impact of AIDS on Gay Male Sexual Behaviour Patterns in New York City*, *American Journal of Public Health*, 77, pp. 578–581.

MASTERS, W.H. and JOHNSON, V.E. (1979) *Homosexuality in Perspective*, Little, Brown & Co, New York.

Maupin, A. (1984) *Further Tales of the City*, Corgi, London.

Mayer, K.H., Ayotte, D., Groopman, J.E., Stoddard, A.M., Sarngadharan, M. and Gallo, R. (1986) 'Association of Human T Lymphotropic Virus Type III Antibodies with Sexual and Other Behaviours in a Cohort of Homosexual Men With and Without Generalised Lymphadenopathy', *American Journal of Medicine*, 80, pp. 357–363.

McCusker, J., Stoddard, A.M., Mayer, K.H., Cowan, D.N. and Groopman, J.E. (1988) 'Behavioural Risk Factors for HIV Infection among Homosexual Men at a Boston Community Health Center', *American Journal of Public Health*, 78, 1, pp. 68–71.

McIntosh, M. (1968) 'The Homosexual Role', *Social Problems*, 16, 2, reprinted in Plummer, K. (Ed.), (1981) *The Making of the Modern Homosexual*, Hutchinson, London, and more recently in Stein, E. (1991) *Forms of Desire*, Routledge, London, pp. 25–42.

McKegany, N. (1992) 'Hooked on the Killing Game', *The Times Higher Education Supplement*, July 3, p. 17.

McKirnan, D., Doll, L., Harrison, J., Delagdo, W., Doetsch, J., Mendoza, G. and Burzette, R. (1991) *Primary Relationships Confer Risk for HIV Exposure among Gay Men*, poster presented at VIIth International Conference on AIDS, Florence, MD4049.

McKusick, L., Coates, T.J., Morin, S.F., Pollack, L. and Hoff, C. (1990) 'Longitudinal Predictors of Reductions in Unprotected Anal Intercourse Among Gay Men in San Francisco', *American Journal of Public Health*, 80, 8, pp. 978–983.

McManus, T.J. and McEvoy, M. (1987) 'Some Aspects of Male Homosexual Behaviour in the UK: a Preliminary Study', *British Journal of Sexual Medicine*, April.

McKusick, L., Hartman, W. and Coates, T.J. (1987) *Prevention of HIV Infection Among Gay and Bisexual Men: Analysis of Two Longitudinal Studies*, Paper presented at the III International Conference on AIDS, Washington, DC.

McKusick, L., Hartman, W. and Coates, T.J. (1985) 'AIDS and Sexual Behaviour Reported by Gay Men in San Francisco', *American Journal of Public Health*, 75, pp. 493–496.

McWhirter, D.P. and Mattison, A.M. (1984) *The Male Couple: How Relationships Develop*, Prentice-Hall, Englewood Cliffs, NJ.

Melbye, M., Biggar, R.J., Ebbesen, P., Sarngadharan, M.G., Ayotte, D., DeVico, A.L., Finberg, R., Sliski, A.H., Allan, J.D. and Gallo, R.C. (1984) 'Seroepidemiology of HTLV-III Antibody in Danish Homosexual Men: Prevalence, Transmission, and Disease Outcome', *British Medical Journal*, 289, pp. 573–575.

Mendola, M. (1980) *The Mendola Report: A New Look at Gay Couples in America*, Crown Publishers, New York.

Millett, K. (1969) *Sexual Politics*, American edition, Avon, New York.

Morin, J. (1986) *Anal Pleasure and Health*, Yes Press, Burlingame, CA, (2nd edition).

Moss, A.R., Osmond, D., Bacchetti, P., Chermann, J.C., Barre-Sinoussi, F. and Carlson, J. (1987) 'Risk Factors for AIDS and HIV Seropositivity in Homosexual Men', *American Journal of Epidemiology*, 125, 6, pp. 1035–1047.

MURRAY, S.O. (1992) 'The "Underdevelopment" of Modern/Gay Homosexuality in Meso-America', in PLUMMER, K. (Ed.) *Modern Homosexualities: Fragments of a Gay and Lesbian Experience*, Routledge, London, pp. 29–38.

NICHOLS, E.K. (1989) *Mobilizing Against AIDS* (2nd edition), Harvard University Press, London.

NICHOLSON, J.K.A., MCDOUGAL, J.S. and JAFFE, H.W. *et al.* (1985) 'Exposure to Human T-Lymphotropic Virus Type III/Lymphadenopathy-Associated Virus and Imunological Abnormalities in Asymptomatic Homosexual Men', *Annals of Internal Medicine*, 103, pp. 37–42.

NORTON, R. (1992) *Mother Clap's Molly House: Gay Subculture in England 1700–1830*, Gay Men's Press, London.

ODETS, W.W. (1992) 'Unconscious Motivations for the Practice of Unsafe Sex among Gay Men in the United States', Poster presented at the VIII International AIDS Conference, Amsterdam, PoD 5191.

OSMOND, D., BACCHETTI, P., CHAISSON, R.E., KELLY, T., STEMPEL, R., CARLSON, J. and MOSS, A.R. (1988) 'Time Exposure and Risk of HIV Infection in Homosexual Partners of Men with AIDS', *American Journal of Public Health*, 78, 8, pp. 944–948.

PADIAN, N., MARQUIS, L. and FRANCIS, D. *et al.* (1987) 'Male to Female Transmission of Human Immunodeficiency Virus', *Journal of the American Medical Association*, 258, pp. 788–791.

PARKER, R. (1987) 'Acquired Immunodeficiency Syndrome in Urban Brazil', *Medical Anthropology Quarterly*, 1, 2, pp. 155–175.

PARRY, J.V. (1986) 'An Immunoglobin G Capture Assay (GACRIA) for Anti-HTLV III/LAV and Its Use as a Confirmatory Test', *Journal of Medical Virology*, 19, pp. 387–397.

PARRY, J.V., PERRY, K.R. and MORTIMER, P.P. (1987) 'Sensitive Assays for Viral Antibodies in saliva; an Alternative to Tests on Serum', *Lancet*, ii, pp. 72–5.

PATTON, C. (1985) *Sex and Germs: The Politics of AIDS*, South End Press, Boston, MA.

PEPLAU, L.A. and COCHRAN, S. (1981) 'Value Orientation in the Intimate Relationships of Gay Men', *Journal of Homosexuality*, 6, pp. 1–19.

PEPLAU, L.A. (1981) 'What Homosexuals Want in Relationships', *Psychology Today*, 15, pp. 28–38.

PLUMMER, K. (1988) 'Organising AIDS', in AGGLETON, P. and HOMANS, H. *Social Aspects of AIDS*, Falmer Press, London, pp. 20–51.

PLUMMER, K. (1975) *Sexual Stigma: An Interactionist Account*, Routledge Kegan Paul, Boston, MA.

PLUMMER, D. (1963) *Queer People*, W.H. Allen, London.

POLLAK, M. (1988) *Les Homosexuels et le SIDA: Sociologie d'une Épidémie*, AM Métailié, Paris.

POLLAK, M. (1992) 'Assessing AIDS Prevention Among Male Homo- and Bisexuals', in PACCAUD, F., VADER, J.P. and GUTZWILLER, F. (Eds), *Assessing AIDS Prevention*, Birkhauser Verlag, Basel.

POMEROY, W.B. (1972) *Dr. Kinsey and the Institute for Sex Research*, Nelson, New York.

PONTE, M.R. (1974) 'Life in a Parking Lot: An Ethnography of a Homosexual Drive-in', in JACOB, J. (Ed.), *Field Studies and Self Disclosures*, National, California.

Porter, K. and Weeks, J. (Eds) (1990) *Between the Acts: Lives of Homosexual Men 1885–1967*, Routledge, London.

Powell, E.J. (1988) *The Feminine in the Thought of Martin Buber*, Unpublished Ph.D. Thesis, University of Wales.

Prieur, A. (1990) 'Gay Men: Reasons for Continued Practice of Unsafe Sex', *AIDS Education and Prevention*, 2, 2, pp. 110–117.

Ramey, J.W. (1975) 'Intimate Groups and Networks: Frequent Consequences of Sexually Open Marriages', *Family Coordinator*, 24, 5, pp. 15–30.

Read, K.E. (1980) *Other Voices: The Style of a Male Homosexual Tavern*, Chandler & Sharp, Novato NY.

Richardson, D. (1990) 'AIDS Education and Women: Sexual and Reproductive Issues', in Aggleton, P., Davies, P.M. and Hart, G. (Eds), *AIDS: Individual, Cultural and Policy Dimensions*, Falmer Press, London, pp. 169–79.

Robertson, H. (1988) 'AIDS: A Trade Union Issue', in Aggleton, P. and Homans, H. (Eds), *Social Aspects of AIDS*, Falmer Press, London.

Ross, M.W. (1988) 'Attitudes Toward Condoms as AIDS Prophylaxis in Homosexual Men: Dimensions and Measurement', *Psychology and Health*, 2, pp. 291–99.

Ross, M.W. (1990) 'Married Homosexual Men: Prevalence and Background', *Marital and Family Studies*, pp. 35–37.

Ross, M.W. (1988) 'Personality Factors that Differentiate Homosexual Men with Positive and Negative Attitudes toward Condom Use', *New York State Journal of Medicine*, pp. 626–28.

Rotter, J.B. (1966) 'Generalised Expectancies for Internal Versus External Control of Reinforcement', *Psychological Monographs*, 80, 1, pp. 1–26.

Rowbotham, S. and Weeks, J. (1977) *Socialism and the New Life: The Personal and Sexual Politics of Edward Carpenter and Havelock Ellis*, Pluto Press, New York.

Rumaker, M. (1978) *A Day and a Night at the Baths*, Grey Fox, San Francisco.

Ruse, M. (1988) *Homosexuality: A Philosophical Enquiry*, Blackwell, Oxford.

Saghir, M.T. and Robins, E. (1973) *Male and Female Homosexuality — A Comprehensive Investigation*, The Williams and Wilkins Company, Baltimore.

Salzman, S.P. *et al.* (1987) 'Reliability of Self-reported Sexual Behaviour Risk Factors for HIV Infection in Homosexual Men', *Public Health Reports*, 102, 6, pp. 692–7.

Sasse, H., Bigagli, A., Chiarotti, F., Martucci, P., Greco, D. and Grillini, F. (1991) 'Homosexual Practices with Steady and Non-Steady Partners among Men Frequenting Public Gay Meeting Places in Italy', poster presented at VIIth International Conference on AIDS, Florence, WC3011.

Schechter, M.T., Boyko, W.J., Douglas, B. *et al.* (1986) 'The Vancouver Lymphadenopathy-AIDS Study: 6. HIV Seroconversion in a Cohort of Homosexual Men', *Canadian Medical Association Journal*, 135, pp. 1355–1360.

Schmidt, K.W., Fouchard, J.R., Krasnik, A., Zoffman, H., Jocobsen, H.L. and Kreiner, S. (1992) 'Sexual Behaviour Related to Psycho-Social Factors in a Population of Danish Homosexual and Bisexual Men', *Social Science and Medicine*, 34, 10, pp. 1119–1127.

Schofield, M. (1965) *Sociological Aspects of Homosexuality: A Comparative Study of Three Types of Homosexual*, Longmans, London.

Schofield, M. (1965) *The Sexual Behaviour of Young People*, Longmans, Green & Co., London.

SCHRAMM EVANS, Z. (1990) 'Responses to AIDS, 1986–1987', in AGGLETON, P., DAVIES, P.M. and HART, G. (Eds), *AIDS: Individual, Cultural and Policy Dimensions*, Falmer Press, London, pp. 221–32.

SCOTT, P. (1992) 'National AIDS Manual', NAM Publications, London.

SEABROOK, J. (1976) *A Lasting Relationship: Homosexuals and Society*, Allen Lane, London.

SEDGEWICK, E.K. (1990) *Epistemology of the Closet*, New York, Harvester Wheatsheaf.

SELIGMAN, M.E.P. (1975) *Helplessness: On Depression, Development and Death*, Freeman, San Francisco.

SEXUAL OFFENCES BILL 1967 (UK)

SHERR, L. (1990) 'Fear, Arousal and AIDS: Do Shock Tactics Work?' *AIDS*, 4, pp. 361–4.

SHILTS, R. (1987) *And the Band Played On: People, Politics and the AIDS Crisis*, Penguin, London.

SIEGAL, F.P. and SIEGAL, M. (1983) *AIDS: The Medical Mystery*, Grove Press, New York.

SIEGEL, K., MESAGNO, F., CHEN, J.Y. and CHRIST, G. (1989) 'Factors Distinguishing Homosexual males Practicing Risky and Safer Sex', *Social Science and Medicine*, 28, 6, pp. 561–569.

SONTAG, S. (1988) *AIDS and Its Metaphors*. Penguin Books, Harmondsworth.

SONTAG, S. (1978) *Illness as Metaphor*, Straus & Giroux, New York.

SOSKOLNE, V., BENTWICH, Z. and ALMOG, N. (1991) 'Distribution and Determinants of High Risk Behaviour among Homosexual and Bisexual Men in Israel', Poster presented at VII International Conference on AIDS, Florence, M.D. 4705.

SPADA, J. (1979) *The Spada Report: The Newest Survey of Gay Male Sexuality*, Signet Books, New York.

STAINTON-ROGERS, W. (1991) *Explaining Health and Illness*, Harvester Wheatsheaf, London.

STALL, R.D. (1988) 'The Prevention of HIV Infection Associated with Drug and Alcohol Use During Sexual Activity', in SOIEGEL, L. (Ed.), (1988) *AIDS and Substance Abuse*, Harrington, New York, pp. 73–88.

STEVENS, C.E., TAYLOR, P.E., ZANG, E.A., MORRISON, J.M., HARLEY, E.J., RODRIGUEZ DE CORDOBA, S., BACINO, C., TING, R.C.Y., BODNER, A.J., SARNGADHARAN, M.G., GALLO, R.C. and RUBENSTEIN, P. (1986) 'Human T-cell Lymphotropic Virus Type III Infection in a Cohort of Homosexual Men in New York City', *Journal of the American Medical Association*, 255, pp. 2167–2172.

STRONG, P. and BERRIDGE, V. (1990) 'No One Knew Anything: Some Issues in British AIDS Policy', in AGGLETON, P., DAVIES, P.M. and HART, G. (Eds) (1990) *AIDS: Individual, Cultural and Policy Dimensions*, Falmer Press, London, pp. 233–52.

STYLES, J. (1979) 'Insider/Outsider: Researching Gay Baths', *Urban Life 1979*, 8, pp. 135–52.

SYMONDS, J.A. (1983) *Male Love: A Problem in Greek Ethics and Other Writings* (Ed. LAURITSEN, J.), Pagan Press, New York.

TAPINC, H. (1992) 'Masculinity, Femininity and Turkish Male Homosexuality', in PLUMMER, K. (Ed.) *Modern Homosexualitites: Fragments of a Gay and Lesbian Experience*, Routledge, London, pp. 39–52.

TATCHELL, P. (1986) *Aids: A Guide to Survival*, Gay Men's Press, London.

THEWELEIT, K. (1989) *Male Bodies: Psychoanalysing the White Terror (Male Fantasies, volume II)*, Blackwell, Oxford.

THOMSON, R. and SCOTT, S. (1991) *Learning About Sex: Young Women and the Social Construction of Sexual Identity*, WRAP Working Paper 4, Tufnell Press, London.

THT STATISTICS BRIEFING (1992) *HIV and AIDS Statistics to the End of September 1992*, (Terrence Higgins Trust Statistics Briefing Team: DEANE, T., KUTLER, C. and KAHN, M.), October 30th.

TRIPP, C.A. (1975) *The Homosexual Matrix*, Signet, New York.

TROIDEN, R.R. and GOODE, E. (1975) 'Homosexual Encounters in a Highway Rest Stop', in GOODE, E. and TROIDEN, R.R. (Eds), *Sexual Deviance and Sexual Deviants*, William Morrow, New York.

TROIDEN, R.R. (1988) 'Homosexual Identity Development', *Journal of Adolescent Health Care*, 9, pp. 105–113.

TURNER, B. (1984) *The Body and Society*, Blackwell, Oxford.

TVERSKY, A. and KAHNEMAN, D. (1974) *Judgement Under Uncertainty: Heuristics and Biases*, Science, 185, pp. 1124–1131.

VAN GRIENSVEN, J.P.G., DE VROOME, E.M.M., GOUDSMIT, J. and COUTINHO, R.A. (1989) 'Changes in Sexual Behaviour and the Fall in Incidence of HIV Infection Among Homosexual Men', *BMJ*, 298, pp. 218–221.

VAN GRIENSVEN, J.P.G., TIELMAN, R.A.P., GOUDSMIT, J., VAN DER NOORDAA, J., DE WOLF, F., DE VROOME, M.M. and COUTINHO, R.A. (1987) 'Risk Factors and Prevelance of HIV Antibodies in Homosexual Men in the Netherlands', *American Journal of Epidemiology*, 125, 6, pp. 1048–1057.

VAN DE PERRE, P., JACOBS, D. and SPRECHER-GOLDBERGER, S. (1989) 'The Latex Condom, an Efficient Barrier Against Sexual Transmission of AIDS-Related Viruses', *AIDS*, 1, pp. 49–52.

VASS, A.A. (1986) *AIDS: A Plague In Us*, Venus Academica, St. Ives, Cornwall.

WARREN, C.A.B. (1974) *Identity and Community in the Gay World*, Wiley, New York.

WATNEY, S. (1989) 'Taking Liberties: An Introduction', in CARTER, E. and WATNEY, S. (Eds), *Taking Liberties: AIDS and Cultural Politics*, Serpent's Tail, London, pp. 59–68.

WATNEY, S. (1989) 'AIDS, Language and the Third World', in CARTER, E. and WATNEY, S. (Eds), *Taking Liberties: AIDs and Cultural Politics*, Serpent's Tail, London, pp. 183–92.

WATNEY, S. (1989) 'The Subject of AIDS', in AGGLETON, P., DAVIES, P. and HART, G. (Eds), *AIDS: Social Representations, Social Practices*, Falmer Press, London, pp. 64–73.

WATNEY, S. (1987) 'Policing Desire: Pornography, AIDS and the Media', Comedia, London.

WEATHERBURN, P., DAVIES, P.M., HUNT, A.J., COXON, A.P.M. and MCMANUS, T.J. (1990) 'Heterosexual Behaviour in a Large Cohort of Homosexually Active Men in England and Wales', *AIDS Care*, 2, 4, pp. 319–24.

WEATHERBURN, P., HUNT, A.J., DAVIES, P.M., COXON, A.P.M. and MCMANUS, T.J. (1991) 'Condom Use in a Large Cohort of Homosexually Active Men in England and Wales', *AIDS Care*, 3, 1, pp. 31–41.

WEATHERBURN, P. (1990) 'HIV, STDs and Perceived Risk: A Theoretical Overview and Two Pilot Studies', Project SIGMA Working Paper no. 11, London.

WEEKS, J. (1977) *Coming Out: Homosexual Politics in Britain from the Nineteenth Century to the Present*, Quartet, London.

WEEKS, J. (1988) 'AIDS: The Intellectual Agenda', in AGGLETON, P., DAVIES, P. and HART, G. (Eds) *AIDS: Social Representations, Social Practices*, Falmer Press, London, pp. 1–20.

WEINBERG, M.S. and WILLIAMS, C.J. (1974) *Male Homosexuals: Their Problems and Adaptations*, Penguin, New York.

WEINBERG, M.S. and WILLIAMS, C.J. (1975) 'Gay Baths and the Social Organisation of Impersonal Sex', *Social Problems*, 23, pp. 124–36.

WEINBERG, G. (1973) *Society and the Healthy Homosexual*, Anchor, Garden City, New York.

WEINBERG, T.S. (1978) 'On "Doing" and "Being" Gay: Sexual Behaviour and Homosexual Male Self-Identity', *Journal of Homosexuality*, 4, 2, pp. 143–56.

WEINBERG, M. (1970) 'Homosexual Samples: Differences and Similarities', *Journal of Sex Research*, 6, pp. 312–25.

WELLINGS, K. (1988) 'Perceptions of Risk: Media Treatment of AIDS', in AGGLETON, P. and HOMANS, H. (1988) *Social Aspects of AIDS*, Falmer Press, London, pp. 83–105.

WEST, D.J. (1955) *Homosexuality*, Duckworth, London.

WELLINGS, K., FIELD, J., JOHNSON, A., WADSWORTH, J. and BRADSHAW, S. (1990) 'Notes on the Design and Construction of a National Survey of Sexual Attitudes and Lifestyles', in HUBERT, M. (Ed.) (1990) *Sexual Behaviour and Risks of HIV Infection*, Facultés Universitaires Saint-Louis, Brussels.

WESTWOOD, G. (1960) *A Minority: A Report on the Life of the Male Homosexual in Great Britain*, Longmans, London.

WESTWOOD, G. (1952) *Society and the Homosexual*, Gollancz, London.

WHITEHEAD, T. (1989) 'The Voluntary Sector: Five Years On', in CARTER, E. and WATNEY, S. (Eds), *Taking Liberties: AIDS and Cultural Politics*, Serpent's Tail, London.

WILLIAMSON, J. (1989) 'Every Virus Tells a Story: The Meaning of HIV and AIDS', in CARTER, E. and WATNEY, S. (Eds), *Taking Liberties: AIDS and Cultural Politics*; Serpent's Tail, London, pp. 69–80.

WILSON, P. (1993) 'Transformation of HIV Related Legal Problems in the Voluntary Sector', in AGGLETON, P., DAVIES, P.M. and HART, G. (Eds) *AIDS: The Second Decade*, Falmer Press, London [in press].

WINCH, P. (1958) *The Idea of a Social Science*, RkP, London.

WINKELSTEIN, W., LYMAN, D.M., PADIAN, N., GRANT, R., SAMUEL, M., WILEY, J.A., ANDERSON, R.E., LANG, W., RIGGS, J. and LEVY, J.A. (1987) 'Sexual Practices and Risk of Infection By the Human Immunodeficiency Virus', *Journal of the American Medical Association*, 257, 3, pp. 321–325.

WINKELSTEIN, W., WILEY, J.A., PADIAN, N. and LEVY, J. (1986) 'Potential for Transmission of AIDS-Associated Retrovirus from Bisexual Men in San Francisco to Their Female Sexual Contacts', *Journal of the American Medical Association*, 256, pp. 901.

YOUNG, A. (1973) *Gay Gringo in Brazil*, in *The Gay Liberation Book*, Ramparts Press, San Francisco, pp. 60–67.

Index